LEARNING
TO LIVE WITH IT

By Kevin Olson

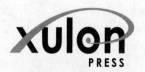

TABLE OF CONTENTS

INTRODUCTION
— JAMES: LIVE WITH IT

I was sitting in the backyard at my mother's house, enjoying the warmth of the summer sun. My youngest brother, James, was playing in the sandbox beneath a nearby maple tree. As I sat there watching him, a bird flew by and pooped on my shoulder. I was a bit disgusted with the bird, yet thankful my head had not been hit.

Immediately I hollered to James, "Come here!" He responded like a typical three-year-old and simply asked, "Why?"

I did not want to tell him, but I did not want to lie either. I knew James loved to help me with things, so I said, "Because I need your help."

He put down his toys, brushed a little sand off, and waddled over to me. I said, "Do you see that stuff there on my shoulder?"

"Yes," he replied.

"Will you wipe it off?"

He reached towards my shoulder, and just when it looked as if he was going to wipe it off, he froze. His eyes met mine, and he said, "Kevin, what is that?"

Hesitantly I said, "Uh, well, a bird flew by and dropped this on my shoulder. I'm pretty sure it's bird poop."

James jerked his hand back, wrinkled up his nose, and exclaimed, "I'm not touching that!"

I knew Mom would help me, so I said, "Then go get Mom."

James looked at me and sternly said, "Okay, but if she doesn't want to wipe it off, then you're just going to have to live with it!"

Mom came out of the house to remove the mess, but my brother's words had penetrated my soul. It seemed as if through him, God was reminding me of one of the first things we learn in this world as children. When we can't change a circumstance, we have to learn to live with it.

At the time this happened, I had been paralyzed for two years. The doctors had said there was no chance I would regain the use of my arms or legs. I had been praying a lot to walk again. I had done everything I knew to do. I had fasted, called for the elders of the church to anoint me with oil, memorized and repeated healing promises from

Scripture, called prayer lines, and even traveled to a healing crusade.

Seeing no physical change did not change my belief that God could heal me, but it was discouraging, and I was struggling to accept *no*. I did not want to learn to live with paralysis. I wanted God to remove my unwanted circumstance so that I could continue living my life as I had planned.

Section 1

MY STORY

For a long time it had seemed to me that life was about to begin—real life. But there was always some obstacle in the way, something to be gotten through first, some unfinished business, time still to be served, a debt to be paid. Then life would begin. At last it dawned on me that these obstacles were my life.

—Alfred D. Souza

Chapter 1

THE CHOICE

Monday, July 15, 1991

I woke to the morning sun peeking over the distant treetops. As I looked eastward, the sun was just beginning to reflect off the water. The lake looked like a big sheet of glass, and no boats were in sight. It was a water skier's dream.

I thought, "This is going to be a perfect day."

The cool morning air surrounding my sleeping bag made me hesitant to uncover, but the hard surface of my pickup bed and the anticipation of a new day won out. I thanked God for giving me this day, tossed aside my blanket, and started moving about the campsite.

Three of my friends and coworkers, Trent, Travis, and Jerrod, had accompanied me to the small Kansas lake the afternoon before. We brought a boat, a jet ski, a motorcycle, two pickup trucks, and just enough necessities for four guys to call it a camping trip.

It had been a good summer. We were working together in the hay fields, as we had for several years, trying to make a little extra money to help with college. Trent was a year older than I and Travis a year younger, but both had started hauling hay with me during high school. They were brothers; both were built pretty solid, had sandy-colored hair, and loved to play football and wrestle. Jerrod and I had played baseball and basketball together since fourth grade. I towered over him in little league, but now he stood six feet two and weighed around two hundred pounds. Together the four of us worked all day under the hot Kansas sun, stacking hay in barns for local farmers and ranchers.

We had a job lined up later that afternoon, so we decided to take advantage of the beautiful morning and ski for a couple of hours. Skiing was a love of mine, and I could do almost anything on skis, but today I was going to do something I had never done before: ski barefoot. In previous attempts, I had never been able to stand on top of the water for more than a split second; however, I knew I could do it. I was nineteen, physically strong, and willing to work hard at it until I succeeded. I could do anything. At least, that's what I thought.

The four of us waded out to the blue deck boat and drove back into a cove on the east side of Toronto Lake. I jumped in, grabbed the rope, put a knee board between my legs, and yelled, "Go!"

The boat lunged forward, and within seconds we were moving at 35 miles per hour. I positioned my feet on the surface of the water, pulled harder on the rope, and raised up off the board. Water was spraying everywhere. I opened my eyes long enough to see myself standing on top of the water. My success was short-lived, but I had done it. I had skied with no skis.

That morning I had no fear of anything. I felt as if I could take on the world and win. I felt invincible, as if nothing could ever happen to me that I couldn't handle.

After a couple of hours of fun on the lake, we beached the boat in front of our campsite and waded ashore. Jerrod and Travis began picking up around the campsite, while Trent and I began wrestling. The winner would drive my pickup to the boat ramp and back the trailer into the water. I won the honors, so he went to load up his jet ski.

As I took off in my dark-blue Chevy Silverado, I was proud of the fact that I had won the wrestling match with Trent, since he was a wrestler and I was a basketball player. (I'm sure he would say he let me win.) However, I had even bigger reasons for being high on life than being able to ski barefoot and outwrestle my friend. I was excited about where my life was headed. I was chasing my dream, and the world was mine for the taking.

My life's dreams weren't outlandish. I had given up on thinking I would one day be in the Major Leagues or the NBA. I wanted to finish college, find a good job, have my own farm, find a wife, and start a family of my own. I was determined to do whatever I needed to do to accomplish these goals, and I was not going to let anything or anyone stand in my way.

Things were moving along. I had graduated from Chanute High School in May of 1989, and my last semester of junior college was set to start in August. I was running my own hay-hauling business, and my grandparents and dad were allowing me to farm a few acres and raise cattle. I had also just met a young, brown-haired, brown-eyed Christian girl who seemed to have just about everything I wanted. We had been on a few dates, and although it was nothing serious, it was a huge part of my dream to find the right one. There was an emptiness in my heart, and I thought it could be filled only by living out my dream with the right person.

After backing the boat trailer into the water, I stepped out of the truck, without my shoes. I began walking up the ramp, trying to decide how to get to the boat. It was still sitting by our campsite, only about two hundred to three hundred feet away.

My plan was to walk down the road I'd just driven to the campsite and wade out to the boat like we had been doing all weekend, but a sharp rock jabbed my foot after only a couple of steps. The sight of the rough, gravelly surface ahead caused me to turn around. I looked towards the boat dock and contemplated swimming to the boat. Walking on the rocks seemed like a painful way to get there, while swimming seemed a fun way to get a little more exercise. I turned and ran down the narrow bridge that led to the dock next to the ramp, never considering the consequences of my choice.

The dock was only a couple of feet above the surface of the water, and it was usually the place where we docked the boat. This weekend, however, we had been loading and unloading at our campsite, and we had not driven the boat close to the dock. As I approached the water, I started running faster, never thinking about what might happen if the water wasn't deep enough.

With my arms stretched out in front of my six-feet, 180-pound body, I dove out away from the dock as far as I could. My plans to swim to the boat—as well as the plans I had for my life—were interrupted by a rock lying on the bottom of the lake.

"Why did I do that?" I wondered, after hearing something crack like a gunshot. Whatever the reason, I began to realize that something was drastically wrong with my body. My arms and legs would not move, and I was struggling to find some way to roll myself over. I kept telling myself I could do it, but thinking I could roll myself over wasn't changing anything.

The messages I was trying to send were not getting from my brain to my arms and legs. There was a sense of urgency when I reached the point where I could not hold my breath any longer. Water rushed in when I opened my mouth to breathe. I was drowning in a couple of feet of muddy water.

It reminded me of how I had felt my senior year when our basketball team lost our last game by one point. With time running out in the fourth quarter, I missed a wide open ten-foot jump shot. Our dream of going to the state tournament—as well as a huge part of my life—was over the second I missed. We had been beaten, and there were no second chances. While underwater, once again time was running out. Only this time it was not just basketball. It was my life.

Those moments in limbo were some of the most memorable yet humbling of my life. The time I had spent with my friends, my brothers, my sister, my mom, my dad, and my grandparents went through my mind first. Time spent going to school and working in the fields just trying to make enough money to get a good start in life flashed by next.

"Is my life really almost over?" I wondered.

If I didn't get help soon, I knew it would be.

Losing my life and being separated from these people and from my dreams seemed like such a high price to pay for such a small decision. It did not seem fair. This was not supposed to be the end.

As thoughts of my life rushed through my mind, water rushed into my mouth and lungs. I knew Trent was loading the jet ski fairly close to where I was, but I did not think he had seen me. The others were over at the campsite. I didn't know if they had seen me dive in, either. Even if they had, were they close enough to reach me in time? There was no way I could yell at them, so in desperation I did the only thing I could. I swallowed my pride, along with one last mouthful of lake water, and I prayed.

To God, I imagine my prayer sounded as if I were begging or as if I were a defense attorney pleading before the judge not to enforce the death penalty. I told God I was young, with a lot of life left to live, and did not want to die. I felt so unworthy to be asking God for anything now.

Much like Trent and I had wrestled over who would drive my truck, God and I had been wrestling for several months. He had been asking me to give Him the driver's seat of my life, but my pride kept me from admitting I needed to make some life changes and give God the wheel. I wanted God in my life, but I wanted Him as my helper. I wanted Him to help me do the things I wanted to do, but I didn't want Him telling me what to do. I was afraid His plans for my life would not match with mine.

Deep down I knew I needed to give Him control of my life, but I thought I would have plenty of time for that later. Just yesterday, at church, I had basically told God there would always be another Sunday for me to consider what He wanted.

The way things looked now, there would never be another Sunday for me.

My spirit leaped within me when I heard the water splashing around me. Trent had watched me dive in and noticed I was lying motionless in the water. Within seconds after I prayed, he jumped in, rolled me over carefully, and held my head and neck stable while Jerrod went to phone the ambulance. The moment I saw the sun and felt air fill my lungs is indescribable. It was almost as though I had died and come back to life. I had given up on the hope of my own abilities being able to save me.

I was still able to breathe on my own and talk when Trent brought me to the surface. The first question I asked was, "Am I paralyzed?" Trent was planning to be a physical therapist and had just completed a course that covered head and neck injuries. I clung to his response of "I don't think so," but my body was numb. I could not tell where my arms and legs were or if I even had any. Travis held on to my feet because I was afraid of having them go under. Back underwater was the last place I wanted to be.

As the small waves sloshed against my face, into my ears, and close to my mouth, I tried to stay calm. The guys kept asking me questions like "Where do you live?" "What is your phone number?" "Who are we?" "What's the square root of pi?" At the time, I thought it was annoying, but they were just trying to keep me awake and alert. They did not want me to quit breathing, and neither did I.

Within forty-five minutes, the ambulance arrived. They slid a backboard under my body, lifted me out of the water, and loaded me into the ambulance. I was still conscious and could talk a little, but my eyes kept rolling back into my head. I had such a headache that I didn't want to open my eyes or talk to anyone. It seemed like too much work.

I spent the afternoon at Neosho Memorial Hospital in Chanute. For most of the few hours, I was in a daze. They took X-rays of my neck, and the doctor said the fifth vertebra was completely shattered. My fourth vertebra was pressing down on top of my sixth vertebra, and my spinal cord was pinched between them. The extent of damage to my spinal cord could not be determined from the X-rays, but the doctor knew I was paralyzed, at least for now.

The nurse asked if I wanted her to call my mom. I said, "No, I'll be fine. She'll just worry."

Over and over I told myself that I would be okay and that I would be able to walk out of the hospital.

Chapter 2

THE CONSEQUENCE

Tuesday, July 16, 1991

What a difference a day makes. I didn't wake up to the sun rising over the lake. I didn't wake up and start moving about the campsite. In fact, I wouldn't even see the sun this day, nor would I move any part of my body except my facial muscles.

My circumstances had changed drastically. Yesterday's excitement about life and what possibilities might be ahead was replaced with worry and fear of what possibilities might lie ahead. I was now a patient at the University of Kansas Medical Center. The only thing that seemed similar to the day before was that when I woke up, I managed to thank God for giving it to me. I was fortunate to be alive.

Twenty-five pounds of weights were fastened to my skull and hung down from the head of the bed. I was in traction, and the doctors were trying to realign my spine before surgery. The doctors and nurses in Kansas City said the same thing as the ones at home: for the moment, I was paralyzed. My family was there in the hospital with me, but there was so much uncertainty. I wasn't really sure why I couldn't move or feel. I had no idea how long I would be paralyzed or how long I would be in the hospital.

At times I was unsure of where my arms and legs were; they often "felt" as if they were floating. At other times, I wasn't sure I even had arms or legs. There was just so much that I didn't know and understand about what was happening to me. How would this affect my life plans? Could it really alter the course of my life as I feared?

For now, I was forced to wait for Friday. On Friday the surgeons would remove the shattered vertebra and build a new one from bone scraped off the front of my hips. There was a great deal of anticipation the next two days because there was hope that the surgery would relieve some of the pressure on the spinal cord. If so, I might get some movement back.

Tuesday, July 16, 1991

The Chanute Tribune

19-Year-Old Serious after Mishap

A swimming accident Monday at Toronto Lake has left a 19-year-old man paralyzed and in serious condition at the University of Kansas Medical Center. Impact from the dive fractured Kevin Olson's neck and caused what appears to be serious damage to his spinal cord. Olson is the son of Dave Olson, Chanute, and Rita Hart, Independence. According to his father, Kevin is currently paralyzed and prognosis is dim for a total recovery and use of his legs.

"It was a very bad fracture, and it damaged his spinal cord," Dave said. "We don't know the extent of the damage to the spinal cord. We are getting to talk to him, but he's in a lot of pain. At this point, they can't give him any strong pain medication because they are afraid it will make him stop breathing."

Olson was flown to Kansas City by Lifeflight helicopter Monday afternoon from Neosho Memorial Hospital where medical officials had listed him in critical condition. Dave said this morning the family was told Kevin was stabilizing, but he remains in serious condition.

"He is in traction, and some of the vertebrae have realigned," Dave said. *Surgery is expected within the next few days to fuse together some of the broken and crushed vertebrae.*

"What Kevin really needs now is everyone's prayers," Dave said. *"We hate to paint a bad picture, but the doctors aren't painting a very good one for us."*

Kevin, a 1989 graduate of Chanute High School, was taking the weekend off from work in the hay fields. The camping trip was spent with friends and co-workers Jerrod Richards, Trent Schell, and Travis Schell, all of Chanute.

They were preparing to leave the lake Monday around 11:30 a.m. and getting ready to remove the boat and jet ski from the water when the accident occurred.

According to Jerrod, "Kevin said he would swim out to retrieve the boat, when he dove off the dock. Then Trent looked over and saw him facedown and saw the blood (from a head laceration). Trent did an excellent job. I'm glad he was there because he knew what to do. He had him supported, and the EMT said that was exactly how Kevin needed to be.

"Kevin spoke to Trent as he turned him over in the water and remained conscious during most of the ordeal. Kevin told him, 'I just couldn't turn over,'" Richards said. *"Travis had his feet*

26

the whole time in the water and he didn't know anyone was holding him. We knew it was shallow, but I didn't think it was only a foot deep by the dock. I've seen people jump off it before, but the water was way down."

In an emotional moment this morning, Dave Olson also gave credit to Trent for saving Kevin's life. "I just want to thank him," Dave said. "He held him in the water; he knew he had a neck injury and knew he couldn't move him. We are grateful to Trent."

Trent, a physical trainer at Kansas State University, has had instruction on the evaluation of orthopedic injury and said this morning he recognized the seriousness of Kevin's condition.

"I had a good idea that that was what happened," Trent said. "I didn't know for certain (of the neck fracture), but it was a good possibility."

Kevin's family is allowed to visit the intensive care unit a few minutes an hour, and Dave said the family appreciates the support already received from the Chanute community.

(Courtesy of *The Chanute Tribune*, Shanna L. Guiot, publisher. All material subject to copyright law.)

Saturday, July 20, 1991

I'm not sure what I expected my life to be like when I woke up the morning after surgery, but I didn't expect this. The only things I could do before surgery, breathe and talk, were no longer possible. A tube was taped to my face. It went up my nose, down the back of my throat, and into my lungs. The tube was attached to a respirator, and it was pumping air into my lungs because I could no longer breathe on my own.

The tube made talking impossible. To communicate with people, I had to have them read my lips. When that didn't work, I had to have them ask me *yes* or *no* questions. If I winked back at them once, it meant yes, and if I winked twice, it meant no. Needless to say, it was extremely frustrating, and I was so disappointed.

There was also a halo vest secured around my chest and shoulders, four screws screwed into my skull, and four metal rods bolted to connect the screws with the vest. Turning my head in either direction was impossible because the halo prevented any movement.

The new vertebrae needed time, eight to twelve weeks, to set up and make my neck stable enough to support my head. Twelve weeks was a long time. Would I be stuck in the hospital the entire time? When could I start talking again? Why could I breathe fine before surgery, but not afterwards?

Saturday, July 20, 1991
The Chanute Tribune
Olson Has Surgery

Kevin Olson underwent four hours of surgery Friday to fuse together vertebrae crushed in a swimming accident Monday at Toronto Lake. Dave Olson telephoned The Tribune Friday with an update on his son's condition.

The surgery began around 12:30 p.m. Friday and was necessary to reposition and fuse crushed vertebrae to put Kevin's neck back in proper alignment. Following the surgery he was placed in a halo neck brace to allow the vertebrae time to heal and to stabilize the injury. He will wear the halo a minimum of 8 to 12 weeks.

Doctors fear the accident could leave Kevin paralyzed from the neck down. Dave said it was too early to discuss whether or not the surgery will relieve any of the paralysis, but the doctors did say there was a ray of hope.

Prior to the surgery the family was allowed to stay in Kevin's room all the time, except during doctors' examinations. Now their visits are limited to 15 minutes every two hours and include only the immediate family.

"It will be three to four days before Kevin will be allowed visitors," Dave said. "And doctors believe he will be moved from intensive care to a regular room by Tuesday.

"He still has a great, positive attitude, and he has shown a great deal of strength so far. He's gotten a lot of emotional strength from seeing his friends. He does appreciate all the cards he has received. His sister and friend ran a string of ribbon through the cards to decorate his room."

(Courtesy of *The Chanute Tribune*, Shanna L. Guiot, publisher. All material subject to copyright law.)

Chapter 3

THE BATTLE INSIDE

Saturday, July 27, 1991

I t had been a little over a week since surgery, and things were not getting better. I wanted off the respirator just as badly as I wanted to get out of bed, so they tried letting me breathe on my own. That night my respirations were over sixty per minute. My lungs were collapsing, and I was panicking. My lungs had filled up with all kinds of bacteria from the lake water, and as a result, I nearly died from pneumonia.

Surviving without help breathing was impossible, so I was connected back to the respirator and put into an air bed that tilted from side to side. The bed totally engulfed my body. It was designed to help keep my lungs from filling with fluid and to provide better protection from skin sores, since all I could do was lie there flat on my back.

The pictures of my spinal cord also came back. It had not been pinched or bruised; it had been completely severed, and there was nothing the doctors could do to fix it. When the doctor came in to tell me the news, he simply explained the situation and concluded with, "Son, you'll never walk again."

I didn't take the news well. It wasn't what I wanted to hear. That night I questioned God and told Him the suffering I was going through was unfair. I wondered, was this my punishment for not listening to God? Or was I simply suffering from the natural consequences of my own bad choice?

On the surface, I was fighting a physical battle that nearly took my life on several occasions, but the real war was being fought on the inside. A part of me just wanted to die. I wanted the suffering to end. The thought of never walking again and never being able to do all the things I dreamed of made me want to give up. If I was going to be permanently paralyzed, did I really even want to live?

Another part of me kept saying I still had a few things to be thankful for. I had family and friends who loved me, I knew God could do things that doctors say is impossible, and I believed God had a purpose for letting me live. I had no idea what that purpose was or where the road I was now traveling would lead, but I was hoping it would lead me back home real soon.

Home for me was located on a gravel road about ten miles southwest of Chanute. My parents had bought a four-hundred-acre farm right after my dad's college graduation in 1974. When we moved into the house that was on the property, I was three years old. My sister, Valerie, was born the next fall, and my brother, Brett, came along five years later.

Our farm home sat in the middle of a tight-knit community of farmers. Everyone knew everyone, and it literally felt as if you were surrounded by family. Many of our neighbors had lived in the area their entire lives. They watched me grow up. Some had watched my parents grow up, as both sets of my grandparents also lived and farmed in this community. My mom grew up just a mile to the north and my dad about four miles west. They met in the same rural school I attended up through eighth grade.

For the biggest share of my childhood, my dad farmed with my mother's dad, Bill Fail. They grew wheat, soybeans, milo, and hay for our cattle. During the late seventies and early eighties, our farm was also home to close to a thousand hogs.

There were always chores to be done: animals to feed and water, fields to till, seeds to sow, and crops to harvest.

I learned to take care of the land, the cattle, and the hogs. I loved it all. Well, all except scraping manure off the mother pigs' cement pads. There were times I did not love that job. I would have rather spent my Saturday mornings at home watching cartoons.

Though there were occasions when I did not want to work, most of the time I wanted to be right in the middle of things, helping as much as possible and trying to be like my dad and grandpa. Seeing my parents and grandparents work day after day to provide for the family left a lasting impression on me. From watching them, I learned that you don't just quit when a job becomes tough or seems overwhelming. You keep working at it little by little. You use your God-given intellect and talents to find a way to persevere and overcome. I also learned there were some things in life you had to do regardless of how you felt and whether you wanted to or not. Lying in a hospital bed quickly became one of those things.

At an early age, I learned how to drive the trucks, the tractors, and the combine. The big machinery was both fascinating and scary to me at first, but I became more confident with experience. A huge wave of self-confidence came over me all about the same time I got my first driver's license and my first real girlfriend. Like any teenager, I thought I was invincible. With confidence came more of a desire to grow up and be independent. With independence came responsibility and freedom.

Most of the time, living under my parents' authority seemed great, but once when I was about ten, I tried running away. For some childish reason, I thought my parents were being unreasonable, so I packed a suitcase and headed out the door to my grandparents' house. I just knew they wouldn't tell Mom where I was. I lugged my suitcase about fifty feet down the driveway and fell flat on the ice. It was freezing cold outside, so I humbled myself real quick and went back inside.

Acknowledging my dependency on them was easy to do at age ten, but now, at nineteen, humbling myself and admitting I needed help from them or anyone else was the hardest thing in the world. However, I had no other choice; it was something I had to do. I thank God for parents who wanted to be there for me at nineteen just as badly as they did when I was ten. Day after day they were there at the hospital for me. When one couldn't be there, the other one was.

I had been a goal-setter for as long as I could remember, and the first goal I set for myself was to walk out of that hospital. Dad had begun teaching me very early that I would never be good at anything unless I worked at it. There were many times we didn't see eye to eye, and there were times when I wished he didn't expect so much out of me. Looking back, I could see that I had learned some of the greatest lessons of life from him.

He pushed me beyond what I thought I could do—and wanted to do—and because of that, I became a stronger person. While lying flat on my back in the hospital, I often thought of the long hours my dad and I had spent playing baseball together in the open space between our green farmhouse and the silver grain bins. I would stand at home plate and swing at pitch after pitch, trying to hit the ball over the grain bins. Then I would play shortstop, and he would hit ground balls towards me over and over until my side hurt so much I couldn't field them.

I thought of the hours we had spent playing basketball in the barn, where my dad hung lights and mounted goals just so I would have a place to play when the weather was bad. I tried to remember how it felt to bounce a cold basketball on the cement floor, the ends of my fingers splitting open because of the cold, dry air and the friction of the ball being pushed away from my fingertips as I shot free throw after free throw.

Life seemed so simple then—no cares, no worries, just sounds of my mom, sister, and brother playing in the yard next to us. Tears would roll from my eyes when I let myself long for the past. I was glad I had not died, but I wanted more. I wanted to go back home and live July 15 over again.

Because I had a tube stuck down my throat, God was the only person I could talk to about how I felt. For a while, it seemed as if He couldn't read my mind any better than my family and friends could read my lips. But one night, as I lay there alone in my room with tears rolling down my cheeks, I felt as if God was saying to me from somewhere within, "Don't give up. Trust Me." So I decided to trust and not give up, to wait and see where this road would lead.

Chapter 4

THE SUPPORT OF OTHERS

Over the next month, news that provided us with a ray of hope would usually be followed by a string of bad news. I say *us* because the fight to move this mountain that had abruptly entered my life had become a team effort. Cards, letters, and donations were coming from people I knew and many I did not. I felt like Glen Campbell must have felt when he wrote the song "Rhinestone Cowboy." As the song says, I was "getting cards and letters from people I don't even know."

Thousands of people showed their concern from a distance, while others were with me, practically living in the waiting room, day after day. I needed their support. Seeing my family and friends was often the only bright spot of my day.

I tried to hide my frustration; I wanted to be strong for everyone else. I was trying to be patient and hoping for the best, but it was tough—tougher than running hours of wind sprints in basketball practice, tougher than getting up every day and going to school, tougher than hauling hay all day, tougher than going through my parents' divorce. It was tougher than anything I had ever experienced.

Monday, July 29, 1991

The Chanute Tribune

Friends Rally to Aid Injured Teen

As friends worked Saturday to raise money for Kevin Olson, the 19-year- old man continues the fight in the University of Kansas pulmonary intensive care unit. Fifteen friends of Kevin's raised more than $1,150 during a car wash Saturday to help the Olson family with some of the pending medical expenses.

This weekend was also a turning point for Kevin as the doctors explained to him his prognosis for the first time. Doctors told Kevin he could possibly develop some use of his biceps, lower arms, and hands, but that was probably all to expect at this time. The doctors also told him not to give up on his hopes and dreams, because that is what makes people go on. Even with a seemingly dim prognosis, Kevin is still keeping a positive attitude and the family is continuing to pray for a miracle.

His muscles have started to contract, and family members continue to work with his arms, legs, and fingers to keep the muscles flexible. He is still experiencing what doctors call "phantom pain" but is now able to receive pain medication. Doctors have said although the pain is not physical, it is very real to Kevin and it will take time for the brain to adjust to the trauma of the injury.

Kevin has reportedly received hundreds of cards from all over southeast Kansas and other states as well. Heather Uden said today that the rain didn't stop patrons who drove through during Saturday's downpour from handing the group donations to the fund. "We'd be standing under the awning, huddled, and people would drive up and say they didn't want their car washed 'but here's 20 bucks,' " she said.

(Courtesy of *The Chanute Tribune*, Shanna L. Guiot, publisher. All material subject to copyright law.)

Wednesday, August 1, 1991
The Kansas City Kansan
Kevin's Accident Meant Abrupt Changes

He was an inspiration to his teammates and a coach's dream. As a high school basketball player, Kevin Olson was dedicated, talented, and committed. A team player.

At Chanute High School he was an All-Southeast Kansas League performer with the sweetest jump shot you could ever want from a shooting guard. I had the privilege of seeing him play many times while covering the Blue Comets as sports editor of The Chanute Tribune. It was a joy to write about this unassuming boy, whose ability and leadership were evident every time he stepped on the court.

That was a couple of years ago.

The other day a friend brought in some recent copies of the Tribune. Everything was great until I scanned the pages, reminiscing about my days in this wonderful small town in southeast Kansas. Then I crossed an article that left a lump in my throat.

Olson, the story read, had been in a diving accident and was paralyzed from the shoulders down. Somehow it didn't seem possible. After all, it seemed like just last week that he was lighting up the gym with his patented jumper, delighting the home crowd. How abruptly things change.

Olson's life is forever changed. The lives of his family members and friends are changed. Business as usual for the rest of us though, right? No. Never has such an incident startled me, forcing a quick assessment of how lucky I am. That's why this is being shared with you through this column.

41

Athletes, especially in high school, rarely take time to appreciate the God-given abilities they have. Actually, most of us probably don't give thanks often enough. It took the tragedy to Olson to make me stop and think about how much I have and how little I take time to truly enjoy it and appreciate it.

Olson was the closest thing to an all-American boy I have ever seen. It appeared there would be no stopping him from succeeding in whatever he chose to do with his life. But his life was altered forever when he dove into shallow water at a nearby lake.

How fragile life is.

(Article by Tom Farmer of *The Kansas City Kansan*)

Thursday, August 2, 1991
The Chanute Tribune
Cards of Support Needed for Olson

For Kevin Olson, cards of support continue to be a source of strength in his hospital room at the University of Kansas Medical Center.

"I want to say that Kevin really does enjoy receiving cards," said his father, David, from the hospital today. "It's really his only entertainment right now."

He noted that the other night Kevin had undergone a minor surgery and physical therapy, so he hadn't had a chance to look at his cards. "It was 10 o'clock, and we couldn't figure out what he wanted. Finally, his sister Valerie figured out he wanted to see his cards. We were up there until 11, reading his cards to him."

David said his son is still on the ventilator, but his pneumonia is clearing up.

"We're glad that he's improving now—the big test will be when they try to take him off the ventilator again, possibly next week. They have begun physical therapy on him, and we're going one step at a time. Trying to get him off the ventilator is the first step."

(Courtesy of *The Chanute Tribune*, Shanna L. Guiot, publisher. All material subject to copyright law.)

Wednesday, August 14, 1991
The Chanute Tribune

Things are looking up a bit for 19-year old Kevin Olson. According to his mother, Rita Hart, Kevin was able to feel a firm squeeze on his elbow this week, which is a welcomed sign that maybe some of the feeling is returning to his upper arms.

The family is taking his recovery one day at a time. He remains in the pulmonary intensive care unit at the University of Kansas Medical Center in Kansas City. Monday he was allowed to eat solid food for the first time since his accident.

"His first meal was mashed potatoes and gravy with meat loaf," Rita said from the family waiting room at the medical center.

In about a week doctors plan to remove the tracheotomy tubing that was implanted to help Kevin breathe during a spell of pneumonia. "As the incision heals, he will begin to talk some," Rita said.

His condition is improving, and only a small portion of the right lung remains affected by the pneumonia. "He'll remain in this ICU until he can remain off the ventilator completely," Rita said. "As far as a time frame, they are not telling us anything. Then he'll move to a regular room, possibly for a week to check his progress, then prepare for a transfer to rehab."

Rita said, "The family is very appreciative of the outpouring of support since Kevin's accident. It's just been tremendous. It not only helps Kevin, but it helps us; it keeps us going. We would not be able to handle it without all our friends. One day we received 63 cards, and it took me an hour to go through them all."

Kevin will celebrate his 20th birthday August 28, and the family is requesting a card shower. Since his accident, local fund-raising activities have been held to boost a rehabilitation account for Kevin.

The family does not want to discourage visitors, but Kevin is still very limited to people he can see, and he gets tired easily.

(Courtesy of *The Chanute Tribune*, Shanna L. Guiot, publisher. All material subject to copyright law.)

Chapter 5

THE UPS AND DOWNS

Wednesday, August 28, 1991

I t was my twentieth birthday. We had cake and ice cream, family and friends were all around, and there were over two hundred birthday cards sent to me; but it was still a somber occasion.

I had been in the hospital for forty-five days, and I was struggling to live with the consequences of my decision. I was still lying flat on my back in the air bed, still had the halo on, and still had a respirator aiding my every breath. There was still no feeling, still no movement, still no shower, and still no verbal communication. Inside I was growing more discouraged. I didn't know how much more I could handle.

Many friends from school and family members were there for my birthday party, but my dad was the one I remember the most vividly. He leaned over my bed, as he had almost every day since July 15, and cried as he tried to mumble *happy birthday*. He didn't have to say anything. The look in his eyes spoke volumes. I knew if there was any way possible, he would take my place in that bed.

He wasn't the only one who struggled with feelings of helplessness. I could see it in the eyes of my mother, my grandparents, my siblings, other family members, and my friends. I could also feel it deep inside my soul.

When I looked into the eyes of my brothers and sister, I felt as though I had let them down. Being the oldest, it seemed my responsibility to teach them to do things like play in the dirt, sort baseball cards, hit baseballs, shoot baskets, work hard, pull pranks on Mom, and make good choices in life. I wanted to be there for them in case they needed me. I wanted them to look to me for strength and help. Now I needed their help.

My twentieth birthday was one of the most depressing days of my life. Memories of past birthdays and thoughts of how much my life had changed kept flooding my mind. The only thing I could see that might be good about this birthday was if God would let me walk again. I wanted my life back. The love and support from family and friends kept me going, but at times it seemed as if I were riding solo in the front seat of a roller coaster that was way off track.

Thursday, August 29, 1991

The Chanute Tribune

Olsons Grateful for Birthday Wishes

Friends, family, and hospital personnel at the University of Kansas Medical Center shared in the 20th birthday of Kevin Olson on Wednesday. Although the celebration was not held under the best circumstances, Kevin's mother, Rita Hart, said today the family is grateful for the birthday cards and well wishes mailed to Kevin.

"Between Tuesday and Wednesday, we received 225 cards," she said. "Cards from all over, from people who hear about him and want us to know he's in their prayers. It's really neat."

Rita said the family has never given up hope, and Kevin is beginning to have "tingling" sensations in his forearms and wrists.

Although the doctors have not removed the tracheotomy implanted to help him breathe during a bout with pneumonia, Kevin has been undergoing 12- to 15-hour breathing trials to keep his lung progress in check.

"He gets along just great in the tests they do after his trials," Rita said. "It's just going to take a while. Day by day it's coming along."

(Courtesy of *The Chanute Tribune*, Shanna L. Guiot, publisher. All material subject to copyright law.)

Thursday, September 5, 1991

Finally, on September 5, I was transferred to a rehabilitation center near Kansas City. It was here that I was able to feel the warmth of the sun on my face for the first time since July 15. Never again would I take that feeling for granted.

The halo vest still restricted me from moving my head, the air bed still engulfed my atrophied body, and my love for hospitals was not growing stronger; yet life was improving gradually. I could talk now and breathe without relying on a machine.

Within hours of arriving there, I met with two therapists whose job was to get my body used to sitting upright again. The first time they tried, I passed out. I was so excited and determined to sit up that when I began to feel light- headed, I didn't tell them. When I woke up, I was lying flat on my back and they were standing around me laughing. Such a simple thing, but my body would have to get used to sitting upright.

For the first time since the accident, I was also able to take a real shower and wash my hair. Putting regular clothes on, feeling clean, and sitting up in a wheelchair gave me a major spirit lift. Talk of getting a chair that I could operate by blowing and sucking on a straw gave me something to look forward to.

Hearing my therapists talk of letting me go home for Christmas motivated me like nothing else could, but I still had a lot to learn. And, in the back of my mind, I still had hopes of beating the odds and walking again.

Saturday, September 7, 1991
The Chanute Tribune
Olson Moves to Rehab

Rita Hart, Olson's mother, said Kevin is expected to be a patient at the Mid-America Rehab Center in Overland Park, Kan., for five months. Although the tracheotomy implant has not been closed, Olson is now completely off the ventilator.

"Little by little he is making progress," she said. "They are working with him to see what he can feel. They said he still has some good muscle in his shoulders, and he can feel down to his elbows now."

Rita said the therapists explained it could take six months to a year for the swelling (around his spinal cord) to go down, and then they will know more of what Olson's limitations will be.

Olson still wears a "halo vest" to support his head, but is now allowed to sit in a chair. The family has been wheeling him in and around the rehab facility.

"He said it felt good to be up. We took him outside, and he said it was good to see the sunshine," said Rita.

(Courtesy of *The Chanute Tribune*, Shanna L. Guiot, publisher. All material subject to copyright law.)

Wednesday, September 25, 1991

After three weeks at rehab, the day finally came when I was able to try driving the sip-and-puff wheelchair I had heard so much about. It was unlike anything I had ever experienced. Blow hard to go forward, blow soft to turn right, suck hard to stop, and suck soft to turn left. For a beginner, I didn't do too badly, but it was the last day I would spend at Mid-America Rehab.

The sensations I was feeling in my upper arms had diminished, and my neck had been causing an unbelievable amount of discomfort. The doctors did not know exactly why. Some thought I just complained so I could get more pain medicine. A CAT scan revealed a possible infection in the bone where they had fused my vertebrae together.

Thursday, September 26, 1991

They loaded me into the ambulance, and I went back to KU Medical Center for an MRI, a high-tech X-ray that takes pictures of internal organs like the spinal cord. When the chief neurosurgeon at KU saw my spine, he immediately scheduled surgery. An infection had invaded the bone that had been placed in my neck during the original surgery to stabilize my spine. They had to remove the infected bone immediately.

The thought of going back to surgery and the possibility of being put back on a respirator made me cry. It seemed as though we were back to square one, starting all over again. However, I couldn't do anything about it; death was my only other option. The screws, bars, and shoulder pads that were placed on me after the first surgery had to come off before another surgery could be done. It was the only positive thing I could think of that came from the news of another surgery.

As the doctor used a half-inch wrench to turn the screws that were embedded in my skull, I shouted, "You're going the wrong way."

He wasn't, but it hurt like nothing I had ever felt. The ends of the screws looked like sharp nails, and the tips were drilled into my skull. One by one they came out, and for the first time in a little over two months, I could turn my head slightly. My neck muscles weren't strong enough to lift my head off the pillow, but at least the halo was gone. The doctors wouldn't promise me it would remain off after surgery, but I sure hoped and prayed it would.

When I opened my eyes after surgery, there were no bars beside my head, no screws in my skull, and no tubes down my throat. I could talk and breathe, thank God. There was more good news too. The infected bone had been completely removed.

The bad news: they had to remove a significant amount of bone, and my neck was no longer stable. There would be no more sitting upright, no more learning to drive a wheelchair, and no trip home anytime soon. I had to wear a neck brace and lie flat on my back for approximately eight weeks. At that point, they would reassess my spinal column and determine whether I needed to repeat the original surgery to re-fuse my vertebrae.

Chapter 6

HITTING ROCK BOTTOM

October 1991

That fall I became a permanent fixture in the neurology wing on the first floor of KU Med. A group of dedicated friends and family continued to show their support, but as time passed, visitors became less frequent. My time alone increased.

Lying there day after day just waiting to get better seemed such a huge waste of time. Floating through life aimlessly without purpose and achievement was not my style. I was always doing something that might get me a little closer to reaching the goals I had set for myself. Now I could do nothing but wait for eight long weeks.

During this time, Kelly, my physical therapist, became like a best friend to me. She had been there since day one and saw my body go from a tan, muscular 180-pound frame to a pale, lifeless 130-pound skeleton. There was no way to keep the muscles from shriveling, but she did come in every morning to move my arms and legs in order to keep the joints from stiffening.

She had just graduated from physical therapy school, and she always came in with a big smile on her face. Some days I would smile back, but there were mornings when I couldn't even open my eyes to look at her. She was close to my age, very pretty, loved sports, and so nice that I would think about my dream of getting married and having a family, then struggle to fight away the tears.

November 1991

Watching old reruns on TV, waiting for more pain medication, and trying to understand just exactly what role God had in all this occupied most of my time. The same questions I had in the first few weeks following the accident kept circulating through my mind. Was this some form of punishment? If so, wasn't this a little much?

I had tons of questions for God. If it wasn't a punishment, why would He allow me to go through this much suffering and disappointment? What was His purpose in this? Or did He even have a purpose in mind?

With each day that passed, the hurt and frustration grew. I was angry with God. I was even angrier with myself. Deep down I knew this was my own fault. God did not make me dive off that dock. Even so, I wanted Him to get me out of this mess.

The days and nights in my room during those eight weeks were some of the loneliest, most depressing times I have ever experienced. It was here that I hit rock bottom. It would almost be winter when the time passed. Waiting eight weeks in bed seemed like torture. I tried not to let anyone see my hurt, but sometimes I just wanted to die. Pain medication seemed my only source of comfort.

Feelings of failure overwhelmed me. I was beginning to understand that my life might never be the same. I was beginning to realize that I might never be able to live out my dreams as I'd hoped. More questions formed in my mind. Would a girl ever want to be a part of my life? Would I be able to have kids? Would I be able to work in any capacity on the farm? If the answer to these questions was *no*, could I ever be content?

I wanted God to come into my room and give me answers, but as it had been since day one, I received no answers. The questions just seemed to bounce right off the ceiling and back into my mind, unanswered. The only thing I heard was that still, quiet voice from somewhere within that kept saying, "Don't give up. Trust Me." I clung to that inner voice, even though I had none of the answers I wanted.

The words *don't give up* reminded me of a poem that hung on a wall in my room when I was a kid. It had often been a source of motivation while I was playing baseball or basketball. The playing field was now different, but the message was the same. This poem, along with the words on a poster that my friend hung in my hospital room, "I can do all things through Christ who strengthens me," kept echoing through my mind.

DON'T QUIT
One of the Hardest Battles of Life Is the Battle Against Ourselves

When things go wrong, as they sometimes will,
When the road you're trudging seems all uphill,
When the funds are low and the debts are high,
And you want to smile, but you have to sigh,
When care is pressing you down a bit
Rest if you must, but don't you quit.

Life is queer with its twists and turns,
As every one of us sometimes learns,

And many a fellow turns about
When he might have won had he stuck it out.
Don't give up though the pace seems slow
You may succeed with another blow.

Often the goal is nearer than
It seems to a faint and faltering man;
Often the struggler has given up
When he might have captured the victor's cup;
And he learned too late when the night came down,
How close he was to the golden crown.

Success is failure turned inside out
The silver tint of the clouds of doubt.
And you never can tell how close you are,
It may be near when it seems afar;
So stick to the fight when you're hardest hit,
It's when things seem worst that you must not quit.

—Author Unknown

Monday, November 25, 1991

The eight weeks had finally passed. The topics of surgery and rehabilitation were once again considered. An opening in Craig Hospital in Englewood (a suburb of Denver), Colorado, and a disagreement over what kind of surgery I needed

58

to stabilize my neck were enough to get me out of Kansas City and on a jet headed for Denver.

Craig was supposedly one of the best rehab hospitals in the world for patients with spinal cord injuries. The move was filled with anticipation, along with a little fear of the unknown. In Denver, I would be ten hours away from family and friends, and there was a whole new set of doctors, nurses, and therapists. I didn't want to go, but I knew it was probably for the best.

Tuesday, November 26, 1991
The Chanute Tribune
Olson Readies for Surgery, Rehab

Tomorrow will be a moving day for 20-year old Chanute resident Kevin Olson. If preparations go as planned, Kevin will be flown from the University of Kansas Medical Center in Kansas City to Craig Hospital in Englewood, Colo., for more surgery and rehabilitation.

According to his father, David, the move is the next step in Kevin's road to recovery. At Craig Hospital, Kevin will undergo an operation to fuse together vertebrae crushed in the accident. The surgery will be performed Dec. 3 and will be similar to the first operation performed at KU on July 19.

"The operation will again align and stabilize the vertebrae," David said. "He's starting all over again. Hopefully this time—with the second fusion surgery—he won't have any complications like he had with the first, like pneumonia and infection.

"He remains determined to come back. He feels he is fortunate to be alive. A lot of things we take for granted, he's grateful for, like being able to breathe on his own. He is in remarkably good spirits. His down times don't last too long."

David said the family is very grateful for the outpouring of concern that has come from the community throughout Kevin's ordeal.

"I want to say thank you to all our friends and to the community for all the support," he said. "That's what has kept us going."

(Courtesy of *The Chanute Tribune*, Shanna L. Guiot, publisher. All material subject to copyright law.)

Chapter 7

MY DAYS AT
CRAIG HOSPITAL

Thursday, November 28, 1991

I arrived at Craig Hospital on the day before Thanksgiving. Dad made the drive out, and we ate Thanksgiving dinner together in my new room. It wasn't at all like Thanksgiving at home. There were no footballs flying through the air, no sounds of laughter and gratitude for God's blessings of health, and no mouth-watering aromas coming from Mom's or Grandma's kitchen.

I did manage to count a few blessings. I could chew the green beans here, and I had roommates who knew what I was going through. Within a couple of days, we also received word that the bone in my neck had grown back enough on its own to support my head. That meant no more surgery and no screws in my skull. For once, it seemed like something had gone right.

December 1991

A few days after Thanksgiving, Dad went home to work. He had started teaching high school math in Chanute and took care of the farm on weekends, evenings, and holidays.

For the next two weeks, Mom and her parents came to be my moral support. My mom had moved to Independence, Kansas, remarried, and had two more boys. Nick was about three, and James turned one during their time with me at Craig Hospital. I watched from a wheelchair as James took his first steps. I remember thinking how ironic that I was watching him learn to walk. I wondered if I would ever learn to walk again.

Physical therapy started right away, but still there was nothing they could do to restore the use of my limbs and nothing to prevent the paralyzed muscles from deteriorating. My neck and shoulder muscles were all that worked, and they were so weak that I could not hold up my head. Being able to hold up my head was a long way from walking, but it was a start, and within a few weeks I could do it.

Occupational therapy was interesting to me because it focused on using the ability I had to become as independent as possible. I met with Christine, my occupational therapist, for one hour each day. She told me from the start that if a positive attitude was all it took to get a paralyzed person up again, then half the patients there would be up running around. She reaffirmed what I had already learned about positive thinking: it has its limitations. However, that did not mean I gave up the hope I had of walking. I let everyone know that if a miracle happened, I would walk the six hundred miles back home.

For now, getting from point A to point B meant learning to blow and suck in a straw that guided an electric wheelchair. I tried out several chairs and put each one to the outdoor test. After getting stuck in the snow and having to be pulled out by my grandpa, a four-wheel drive seemed the logical choice. I wanted to be able to get around on the farm without help. Although there were no four-wheel drives, I picked out one that would go through the grass, the rocks, and a little snow without too much trouble. They began building a chair for me with special seating features so that I could recline and tilt backwards using the sip-and-puff controls.

The stay in Denver went well, but it wasn't without its obstacles to overcome. Less than a month after getting there, I developed a blood clot in my left leg. That meant a week and a half in bed, and it was the worst possible timing. Christmas was coming, and many of my friends and family were going to drive out to see me. In the few weeks at Craig, I had made some positive steps, but now it seemed I would be just like I was in Kansas City—lying in bed, unable to do anything. They would see no progress.

Christmas 1991

I don't remember much about what happened on Christmas Day, but I do remember what I was given. My Christmas gift this year was a trip to watch the Denver Nuggets play basketball against the Boston Celtics. Larry Bird had been one of my boyhood heroes, and I'd always dreamed of watching him play in person. The Celtics were my favorite professional team, but the game was coming up in just a few days. Would the doctors let me out of bed to go?

It had been about ten days since the blood clot was discovered, so after my family learned how to transfer me from a wheelchair into a car, I received permission to go. It was my first time out of a hospital or rehab facility since July 15. I was nothing but skin and bones, and I looked white as a ghost, but I loved it.

When we entered the arena, Scott Hastings, a former Denver Nugget and one of the Nuggets' executives, invited me into the locker room before the game to meet the Denver players. I met basketball greats Walter Davis and Dikembe Mutombo. After the game, they would take us inside the Boston locker room too. I met Larry Bird, Robert Parish, and Kevin McHale. These were guys I had idolized and dreamed about being like as I was growing up. I wondered what they thought as they looked down at me.

January–February 1992

When Christmas passed and everyone went home, it was a lonely time for me, but I knew I had to improve before I could go home to be with my family and friends. Gradually I gained enough endurance to sit in a wheelchair all day, and I learned how to drive through doorways and down hallways without banging into the wall or running into nurses' trays.

Christine made me learn how to drive in the hospital gymnasium for the same reason my dad taught me to drive in the pasture—lots of open space. Learning the difference between a hard puff and a soft puff, a hard suck and a soft suck, was not easy. It took time and a whole lot of practice and patience, but at least I was in control of something, and that felt wonderful.

The sip-and-puff wheelchair was really pretty amazing. It had a long tube that came around my right shoulder and was positioned near my mouth. Blowing hard made my chair go forward, sucking hard made it go backwards, blowing soft made it turn right, and sucking soft made it turn left. When I went forward or backward, the chair would continue without my having to blow or suck. It was like having your car on cruise control. This enabled me to steer while going forward or backward, to increase or decrease my speed, and to stop quickly.

The therapists also taught me how to use a mouth stick. A mouth stick is basically a mouthpiece with a 16- to 24-inch stick attached to it. The end is curved, and it has a rubbery covering on it that resembles a pencil eraser. With the mouth stick, I could write, paint, type, and turn pages in a book.

During these two months, I slowly regained something I had lost—a little independence.

March–April 1992

Freedom came as I learned how to do things. With my wheelchair, I could go places on my own.

With the help of another person, I could leave the hospital. The weekends at Craig were kind of laid-back—no therapy, no classes, and nowhere we had to be by a certain time, except for lunch and dinner. One Sunday after lunch, Brad and I started talking about going to the 7-Eleven store down the street. We often had family and friends go get nachos and drinks, but there was no one around this weekend.

It was nearing spring. We had been inside all winter, and we felt the need to be free. He wanted a pack of cigarettes, and I wanted a Slurpee, so we planned our getaway. It was against hospital regulations to stray from the premises, but we decided to go anyway.

We went down the tunnel that connected Craig with Swedish Medical Center, found the back exit, and headed for the parking garage. The 7-Eleven was just a couple of blocks away, and as long as no one came running after us, we were home free. It wasn't exactly an escape from Alcatraz, but for two guys who had been in the hospital for seven months, it sure felt good.

Brad was a super nice guy, about my age. While driving with some friends, he had flipped his brand-new truck and suffered some severe head injuries. His short-term memory was really bad. He had been in Denver about as long as I had, but his spinal cord had not been damaged like mine, so by this time he had regained a lot of strength. He had progressed from being in a wheelchair all the way up to walking with a walker. Between the two of us, we were almost a complete person. I knew how to get there, and Brad could open the doors and push the buttons on the elevator; and he could also get up the steps and into the store.

The thought of how the two of us must look to people driving down the busy street made me laugh. There I was, blowing and sucking in a tube, rolling down the sidewalk. Brad was limping slowly in front of me, pushing his walker. Every few yards he would stop, turn around, make sure I was coming, and ask which way to go.

When we reached the store, Brad went inside, while I waited in the parking lot. Somewhere along the way, he forgot I wanted a Slurpee, so he bought me a can of Pepsi instead. The nurses always checked the bag that was attached to his walker for things that weren't supposed to be there, so he asked to plant his cigarettes on me. My sweatpants didn't have pockets, so I told Brad to put them just inside my waistband.

We returned undetected. About thirty minutes later, Brad came up to me and said he couldn't remember where he had put his pack of cigarettes.

I told him to look inside my pants, but he objected strongly, saying, "I'm not that kind of guy."

I had to laugh at the situation, but at the same time I thanked God for the ability to think and remember.

Brad wasn't the only one who caused me to feel grateful for what I had. Just a few days before being released to go home, I received a new roommate. About nineteen years earlier, he had been in a bad accident that caused an explosion. Not only was he paralyzed from the waist down, but he was also blind. As I watched him push his wheelchair, feeling his way around the room with his hands, I couldn't help but think how fortunate I was to be able to see.

Looking back over my stay in the hospital, I began to notice a pattern. It seemed that every time I grew discouraged or tried to have a pity party, God would ruin it by showing me things I had to be thankful for.

Chapter 8

NO PLACE LIKE HOME

April 3, 1992

After almost nine months in the hospital, I was dismissed on April 3, 1992. It seemed unbelievable that the day had finally arrived. My dad and my brother Brett flew out and drove my van home.

While I was at the hospital, my family and I had used some of the funds raised by friends and family to purchase a full-size van with a lowered floor and a wheelchair lift. It worked perfectly. I had to ride home in a manual wheelchair, as my sip-and-puff chair was not quite complete. I would need to return to Craig in a few weeks for my chair.

As soon as we pulled onto the entrance ramp of I-70 East, I felt free. Freedom from the wheelchair is what I had longed for, but leaving the hospital would do for now. When I arrived at home that night, there was a welcoming crew hiding in the house. It felt so good to finally be home.

Summer 1992

The first few months at home were tough. It was summertime, my favorite season. Previously summer had meant hard work and lots of fun for me. Besides working in the fields and going to the lake, I had enjoyed hanging out with my friends at night. Sometimes we would play basketball until midnight or sit around on the hoods of our vehicles, just talking.

For most of us, being out of high school meant freedom to go places and do things without asking anyone for permission. Now that freedom was gone. As I watched life go on as usual for my family and friends, I struggled again with the thought of never being able to go places and do things on my own. From the moment I woke up to the moment I went to sleep, and even sometimes in the night, I was always asking for help or needing something done for me.

A typical day used to consist of waking up early, getting ready in a few minutes, and going to school or working on the farm. Now I was forced to wait on someone to come help me out of bed, do my bowel and bladder care, shower me, shave me, brush my teeth, dress me, feed me, give me drinks, and do some range of motion with my arms and legs. Just taking care of the basic necessities to survive and stay healthy took up most of my day.

A handful of friends and family, and a few dedicated caregivers, did everything they could to help me go and do anything my heart desired. Still, I felt trapped in a situation where I had very little control over my own daily activities. It frustrated me to think of spending the rest of my life being dependent on other people.

I felt like a child who needed a cross between a babysitter, a chauffeur, a butler, and a mom. I longed to go to the store, the farm, for a drive, or just go outside my house without having to say a word to anyone about where I was going or why. Being so dependent was not something I enjoyed, but it was something I was going to have to learn to live with and try to make enjoyable for myself and the people who helped me. Ultimately, many of them became close friends.

In many ways, I also became closer to my family than ever before. I moved back in with my dad and often spent the weekends with my mom. My sister and brothers were involved in many sports and school activities. I had plenty of free time to attend. I was so grateful I could still be an influential part of their lives. They loved helping me, and I think I still had a little influence on them because later three of the four chose to go into the medical field. Valerie became a physical therapist and Brett, a physician's assistant. James became a paramedic. Nick became a teacher and coach, but he did work as a caregiver during college.

My grandparents made it a point to visit frequently and did everything they could to involve me in their lives on the farm. My parents were there for me anytime I needed something, often being my most reliable caregivers. Most of my friends were still my friends. Some had gone off to college and work, so we naturally grew apart, but for the most part, nothing changed except the activities we did together. I made a lot of new friends, and I even went out on a few dates.

I never dated any of the girls I went with prior to my accident, but a few visited the hospital and occasionally came by the house to say hello. I was starting to realize that finding the right one to marry might not be as important as I once had thought. I still wanted to find the right one, but it wasn't my number one priority. Figuring out what to do with my life became my main goal.

73

At first, I was unsure of what I could do or where I could go. Talking on the phone, driving my wheelchair, and reading were the only things I could do on my own. A special speakerphone with a sip-and-puff switch was installed by my bed. It had a long flexible arm that mounted to my bed. Inside the arm ran a long tube. Anytime I drove up to the tube and blew in it, the phone would turn on. After five seconds, it would automatically dial 0, and then I would tell the operator the number I wanted to dial. When I was finished talking, I would blow in the tube again and the phone would turn off.

My grandpa built a table that I could drive up to and read from. On it I would have someone place open books, and they would position my mouth-stick holder so that I could grab it with my mouth, then turn pages. Through my teenage years, reading a book was like a form of punishment to me, but now it was one of only a few things I could do on my own, so it soon became something I loved.

The therapists in Denver kept telling me I could find ways to do everything I used to, and to an extent, they were right. However, my life had changed drastically, and there was no way to ignore the fact that I had to live with some major limitations.

The thought of never being able to work on the farm again, never being able to hug someone or hold their hand, and never being able to live out my childhood dreams totally depressed me. Everywhere I went I saw things I could no longer do. After a few weeks of being back in Chanute, riding out to the farm, and trying to figure out what I was going to do with my life, I struggled with feelings of worthlessness. The guys I used to haul hay with were still able to throw bales around, my dad and grandparents were still able to farm, and the work I used to think only I could do was now being done by others.

At night when I lay in bed with the covers up to my neck, I would think, "Well, everything is covered up except the part of me that works."

I often saw myself as nothing more than a spectator in the game of life.

Deep down I knew all of this had happened because I made a bad choice, but couldn't God at least make the consequences a little less severe? I knew He could, but why didn't He? Why had He allowed me to mess my life up so badly?

I found myself back at an all-too-familiar point, a monumental crossroads of sorts that required a decision be made. It was basically the same decision I had been faced with in the hospital, but now I was in a new environment faced with new challenges. Was I going to choose to trust that God had a plan and a purpose for everything He allowed in my life, despite the fact that my life was not turning out like I wanted? Once again, I decided to trust and not give up, to wait and see where this road would lead.

Chapter 9

MAKING THE MOST OF IT

Do what you can with what you have,
right where you are, and don't worry
about the rest.

1992–1994

Since the rehabilitation therapists had encouraged me to do many of the same things I used to do, for the first few years after becoming paralyzed, I managed the hay-hauling business while my friends did the work. I enjoyed this, but at times it was discouraging. Of all the things I missed, being able to work on the farm topped the list. I wanted to be out there sweating under the hot Kansas sun, using my physical abilities to help people and make a living.

I soon discovered that sitting around thinking about all the things I could not do and the things I did not have kept me feeling down, depressed, and discouraged. The more I focused on the things I couldn't do, the more I saw myself as worthless. The truth was, I was not worthless. I just needed to quit looking at all the things I could not do and find things I could do.

Being able to do this required a major change in the way I saw myself. For most of my life, I had used the wrong ruler to measure my self-worth. I saw myself as a useful person, but only because of what I had to give physically. As I looked back on my life, it seemed as if everything I had used to see myself as useful had been stripped from me. When I was twelve, a bad shoulder took a few miles per hour off my fastball and ruined my hopes of playing baseball. In high school, a bad ankle limited my ability to move laterally and jump, so my basketball career ended sooner than I had hoped. My decision to dive off a boat dock at nineteen put an end to working on the farm.

All these circumstances had proven to me that a person's self-worth could not be completely dependent upon their physical abilities. There had to be more. I began to think about what I had to give mentally, emotionally, and spiritually.

I began to try to focus on all the things I could do, instead of the things I could not do.

In the fall of 1992, I enrolled in Neosho Community College to finish my associate's degree. The next spring I graduated. Although I hated speech class, my voice was one of the few things I could use. Mike, a quadriplegic who had done the play-by-play on radio for all my high school games, asked me to do some color commentary during basketball season. Invitations to speak at churches and schools began coming my way also.

I planned to finish college at a four-year school, but I wasn't sure what I wanted to do (or what I could do). As a result of the things I had been through, I was starting to see life as a fragile gift that could be taken away at any moment. There was no guarantee that I would live to be eighty and have the opportunity to do everything I dreamed of. There was no guarantee I'd live to see tomorrow. I wanted and needed something more than what living out my dreams had to offer. I needed something that no person or circumstance—not even death—could ever rob me of.

These things led me to enroll in correspondence courses from Moody Bible Institute in Chicago. As I read and studied the Bible and other books like *When God Doesn't Make Sense* by Dr. James Dobson, I was amazed at what I discovered.

As a kid, I had often thought of the people in the Bible as superheroes and that their lives were free from struggles because God was on their side. As I studied, I realized this was not true. The men and women God worked through in the Bible to do great things were a lot like me. They committed sins that were just as bad as or worse than mine. They were faced with unwanted circumstances that they could not change or understand. During the midst of their struggles, they had to make the same choice I had to make: to trust God or not.

Through their life stories, I saw how in many cases God used their failures and unwanted circumstances to make them stronger and cause their faith to grow. I saw how God loved and used them despite their weaknesses and imperfections. I saw how God loved and used them whether their unwanted circumstances were their fault or not.

Understanding these truths changed the course of my life. Maybe God wanted to use my unwanted circumstances for the same purposes. Maybe I didn't need to know all the answers concerning why things happened like they did. Maybe I needed to focus more on how I was going to respond to my unwanted circumstances and let God take care of the outcome.

I began to ask myself, "Am I going to allow my problems to defeat me, or to develop me? Am I going to allow the unwanted events in my life to make me bitter, or use them to make me better?"

I began to ask God what He wanted me to do, instead of asking Him to help me do what I wanted.

1994–2006

God opened many doors for me to work with people and gave me opportunities to do many things. For a few years, I traveled around speaking at churches, schools, and special events. As I traveled and took time to talk to people, it became increasingly clear to me that many of them were also looking at life from places they never expected or wanted to be. Many were struggling to accept their unwanted circumstances just as I was struggling to accept mine. My story seemed to encourage and inspire others, even able-bodied people.

Early in 1995, as I was looking for ways to give back to my community for the overwhelming support they had shown my family and me since July 15, 1991, I met a man named Walter Aday. I had just finished speaking at a men's luncheon when Walter approached me and told me of an after-school program that was opening called the Cherry Street Youth Center. It was going to be a Christian-based center for kids to attend while their parents were still at work.

This seemed the perfect opportunity, as I was hoping to write children's books and the first piece of advice I received was to spend time with kids. Being completely paralyzed in all four limbs, I was not sure what I could do with kids, and neither was the woman in charge; but she agreed to let me come. With a little help, I discovered I could teach classes, lead games, and be a friend and mentor. I felt as if I was exactly where God wanted me.

On our first day, twenty to thirty neighborhood kids piled into a small house after school and participated in activities until their parents picked them up. From day one, we were turning kids away, so we acquired another lot and built two buildings with playgrounds. Within just a few years, over one hundred kids in grades K–5 were coming to the center each day.

During my first few days at the youth center, a fifth-grade teacher at a nearby elementary school asked me if I would work as a tutor in her classroom. From 1995–2005, I tutored several days a week at Alcott Elementary School, helping kids with math, science, computer, and reading. Many of the same kids who attended school at Alcott walked down to Cherry Street after school, so I often spent the entire day with the same kids.

In 1998, another opportunity to work fell into place. A man from a nearby town called to inform me that their church needed a youth minister. He invited me for an interview, and for the next four years (1998–2002), I worked thirty hours a week as a youth minister for both the First Christian and First United Methodist churches of Fredonia, Kansas.

The highlight of this job was definitely the people I met: the kids, their parents, the church members, and the people we met while going places and doing things. We planned mission trips, canoe trips, work projects around town, bake sales, Bible studies, games, and the list could go on and on. Many of the people here became close friends as well.

From the time I started working, it was my goal to work and support myself financially. I still remember receiving a letter from Social Security in 2000 stating I was no longer considered disabled because I was making too much money. I tried walking after reading the letter, but nothing happened.

In all my work, I found a sense of fulfillment. I felt I was right where God wanted me, and I was enjoying every minute of what I was doing. I was building relationships with kids and adults. I was making a difference in their lives.

The busy schedule eventually caught up with me, and I lost a kidney. I knew I needed to slow down and take better care of myself. I kept working at the youth center, but I resigned from the youth minister position and limited my time tutoring at the school. With the extra time at home, I started writing this book and took correspondence courses in computer programming, learning to build websites.

2007

While none of the places God led me to work enabled me to be completely independent financially, my needs were met through the gracious gifts from others, the hard-working American people who contributed to Social Security, and the work I was given. More importantly, my cup overflowed when I considered the blessings He had given me through the opportunity to meet so many people who enriched my life in their own unique ways.

An unexpected blessing of this kind came my way in 2007 when a man named Kurt Nunnenkamp called, asking if I would be interested in building a website for Paradise Adventures, his outfitting and guide business.

The Nunnenkamp family had been friends of my family since the mid- 1900s. They farmed in our rural community, but I never really had the opportunity to get to know them very well. When Kurt called, I agreed to come down and meet with him one night while he and his hunters had dinner. We discussed his website needs, and I agreed to build a site for him. At dinner I sat next to a blind man who had shot a buck earlier that day. He was so excited about his accomplishment.

Later that evening as I was leaving, Kurt asked me if I would be interested in hunting. As a kid, I had been more interested in other sports; but since becoming paralyzed, I could not participate in any of those sports and had mixed emotions while watching them. I enjoyed them, but at the same time I felt sad because I could not participate. I had little hunting experience, but I was inspired by what I had just witnessed, so I said yes to Kurt's offer.

Kurt built a portable hunting blind, while several of his hunting friends donated money to purchase an adaptive device that mounted to my wheelchair. The device held my gun while allowing me to move the gun in all four directions with a chin-controlled joystick. A sip-and-puff switch was mounted next to the joystick so I could "pull" the trigger.

On my first outing, I shot a turkey. Later that year, I would shoot my first deer. For the first time in years, I was actively participating in a sport, and it felt great. I was more than just a spectator.

Chapter 10

LOOKING BACK

2008–2013

At the time of this writing, I am working from home part-time, creating and updating websites for businesses and organizations. I enjoy being able to help other people grow their businesses, and I've seen my own grow a little as well. I still have the opportunity to travel and speak at schools, churches, and organizations. I've been blessed many times over with the opportunity to encourage and inspire others.

I also still work at Cherry Street. I've worked at the youth center since the day it opened in May of 1995. Over the years, I've taught kids Bible, character development, basketball, games, computers, and many other things. The most rewarding of them has been teaching gardening.

Since the beginning of Cherry Street, Walter had a vision of starting a gardening project with the kids. In 2006, it came to pass, and now we teach the kids how to grow a traditional vegetable garden. They learn the basics about plants and how to care for them. We grow corn, cucumbers, potatoes, onions, lettuce, radishes, peppers, tomatoes, green beans, and sweet potatoes. We've also grown peanuts, strawberries, pumpkins, and watermelons.

The kids are involved in the entire gardening process, from preparing to plant to harvesting. Once a year we set up a vegetable stand and hold a produce sale. We also give produce to the kids to take home, and sometimes we even teach them how to cook what they've grown. The kids enjoy harvesting their produce, while the farm boy inside me enjoys helping them plant something in the ground and watching it grow.

Our vision for the future involves expanding our gardening program to include other methods of gardening with various groups of people, such as at-risk kids and those with limited abilities.

In many ways, I feel like I've accomplished a lot since that life-changing day in July of 1991, and I hope there is much more in my future. But I did not write this book to simply share what I have done. It was written to share the real miracle, what God has done in me.

From where I sit today, I am forced to look at life from a place I never expected or wanted to be—totally paralyzed from the shoulders down, sitting in a chair that I drive by blowing and sucking in a straw, typing this book one letter at a time with a mouth stick. I never wanted to be here. I never wanted to be in a wheelchair, and I never wanted to be a writer.

If you would have told me twenty years ago that I would be able to live a fulfilling life even though I am in this place, I would have told you that you were crazy. As time passed and I looked at my life, I realized that I was going to have to make another choice. This choice has quite possibly been just as influential as the choice I made on July 15, 1991, to dive off that boat dock.

Do I find a way to live with my unwanted circumstances or not?

When I think back on James's words—"You're just going to have to live with it"—I realize they changed the course of my life also. They helped me accept being paralyzed. Eventually the words *live with it* took on another meaning as well. Living with it not only meant accepting the unwanted circumstance, but it also meant finding a way to live life to the fullest despite the unwanted circumstance.

I often wonder where I would be had I not been able to learn to "live with it." I know I would not be here writing and you wouldn't be reading this book, but I really don't know what my life would have been like. I probably don't want to know. Learning to live with it was not an easy choice to make, but it seemed the right choice. I believe that choice has had a major impact on my life and the lives of my family and friends.

As I travel around speaking, I've discovered unwanted circumstances present themselves in all shapes and sizes to all kinds of people. I find many people struggling with their own set of problems, asking God the same kinds of questions I asked, searching for answers.

In the next few chapters, you will find many individual short stories and devotionals that I've written over the years. These stories tell how a combination of people, life experiences, and some truths from God's Word have worked together to help me learn to "live with it" by learning to see things differently.

Section 2

FROM WHERE I SIT

*What happens in you is more important
than what happens to you.*

T he word *outlook* is defined as a view from a
particular place. It usually makes me think
of being in a high place looking out over a beautiful valley, a canyon, or a body of water, but an
outlook is not limited to how we see something
from a physical place on the planet. We look at
every circumstance, person, and event from
wherever we happen to be in life, whether it be
a physical, mental, emotional, or spiritual place.
Simply put, our outlook is the way we see things
from wherever we happen to be.

Chapter 11

BIG THINGS FROM LITTLE PEOPLE

My high school English teacher always told me I should be a writer. I thought she was crazy. At sixteen, I couldn't sit still long enough to read a book, let alone write one. But that was then. . . .

The desire to write a book began to burn inside me about two years after becoming paralyzed. At the time, I thought I wanted to write children's books. While at a writer's conference in Kansas City, I learned that if I wanted to write for children, I needed to spend time with them. I needed to find out what they like, how they think, and the way they learn.

For the next eighteen years, I worked with kids of all ages in after-school programs, churches, and schools. I hung out with them and tried to pay attention to the way they saw life. Little did I know God would use them to change the way I saw mine.

Alicia – Give What You Have to Give

It was a struggle learning to live with paralysis. Not only could I do very little for myself, but I also felt I could do so little for other people. This bothered me because I felt I had nothing to give to anyone. I had always based my self-worth on what I could do physically for myself and for others.

During my third summer at home, I rolled down the street to the city pool. My mission was to give out flyers telling about a Bible school we were hosting at church. While I was sitting by the pool, the cutest little eight-year- old girl I had ever seen came walking up to me. She had brown eyes, brown hair, and a smile that made me feel blessed to be alive.

Alicia stood beside me, talking, asking questions, and smiling from ear to ear. We talked for thirty minutes; then she jumped back into the water. I watched as she swam and splashed, but then I looked away to talk to some other kids. When I turned back, she had disappeared. Next thing I knew, Alicia stood beside me, smiling. She had that I'm-up-to-something look on her face.

She had slipped a Butterfinger onto the armrest of my wheelchair.

As she ate her own Butterfinger, she seemed to realize I needed help to eat mine.

"Do you want me to feed you?" she asked.

"That would be great," I replied.

Fortunately, I love Butterfingers, but for her, I think I would have eaten a can of worms. I'll never forget how special I felt to know that Alicia willingly took some of the money she had been given and used it for me, knowing she would never get it back.

I went home feeling blessed to be alive. Alicia had unknowingly proven to me that life's greatest gifts are often the small things and that giving what I had to give was more important than what I had to give. I couldn't give much to others physically, but I could give to others mentally, emotionally, and spiritually.

Miranda – Look Beyond Your Limitations

Although I could never be used for the things I once took so much pride in doing, and often saw myself as worthless, the truth was, I was not worthless. I just needed to stop focusing on all the things I could not do and look for things I could do.

During my first year tutoring fifth-graders, I met Miranda. Miranda had a cute little smile and the biggest heart in town. She also had a sense of humor and a unique way of looking at things.

For her science project, she and I decided to make a solar cooker out of a cylinder-shaped Quaker-oatmeal container. She cut one side of the container off, leaving the two ends and about two-thirds of the body intact. On the inside, she lined it with aluminum foil; and on the center of each end, she poked a hole just big enough to stick a wire through.

For several days, we loaded the cooker with hot dogs and marshmallows. We kept track of the temperature outside, the amount of sunshine, and the time it took to "brown" our hot dogs or melt our marshmallows. We tried cooking with no lid on our oven versus cooking with a lid. Toward the end, we even added a thermometer to record the temperature inside the oven.

As Miranda became comfortable around me, she said and did whatever came to mind without fear that I would be offended. I liked that because I didn't want kids to feel uncomfortable around me. I wanted them to see that although I had physical limitations, I was just a normal guy.

One day while we were working on her project, the wind blew Miranda's papers everywhere. I felt helpless as I watched her hurry around the yard picking up papers. She ran back towards me, picked up my hand, and put all her papers underneath it. With a sheepish grin, she said, "You make a good paperweight."

Finding things I was useful for became a fun game we played the rest of the year. She discovered my lap made a good shopping cart to carry all her stuff. My feet made a doorstop when nothing else would hold the door open.

This was my first experience working with a child on a science project, but we were both rewarded. Miranda earned a gold medal in the science fair, and I learned that if I would look beyond my physical limitations, I could find many new ways to be useful.

Sierra – Trust God Even When You Don't Know Where He Is Taking You

One positive thing I could see from being paralyzed was that in many cases it actually helped me build relationships with the kids. They were curious to know why I couldn't feel them touching my arms or legs. Seems like I answered the question, can you feel this? a half million times. They were also fascinated by how I could blow and suck in a straw to make my wheelchair move.

They were even more interested when I started giving them rides on the back.

The driveway at Cherry Street was no more than seventy feet long, but long enough to go full speed and give the kids a wild ride. For each passenger, I drove at top speed toward the chain-link gate at the end of the drive. When I reached the gate, I would suck on my straw to stop, then turn around and drive back to where we had begun.

One day as I was giving rides, a kindergarten girl starting running towards me from across the playground. She obviously thought riding on my chair looked like fun, but she didn't know my rules. I allowed only one rider at a time, and everyone had to wait in line. The girl on the back, Sierra, was older and knew my rules; so when the younger girl got close, Sierra stiff-armed her. I should have stopped or slowed down, but I didn't. I kept going.

When I reached the gate, I sucked on my straw to stop, but nothing happened. My feet hit the gate, it swung open, and we headed for the street. I didn't realize it, but while reaching for my chair, the younger girl had grabbed the tube that connects the small computer to my driving straw and pulled it off.

Sierra used to sneak up behind me and turn my wheelchair off just for fun, so I hollered, "Turn the chair off! I can't stop."

It was April 1. She thought I was April-fooling her. I panicked when I realized she didn't believe me. My mother had taught me to look both ways before crossing the street, so I did. I thanked God no one was coming, then swallowed hard. I had no control over where we were going.

Instead of going straight across the street and hitting the curb, my chair started turning slowly to the right. I looked all around for padded walls or giant marshmallows, but the street was lined with cement curbs and vehicles. The only way we were going to stop was to crash, and at full speed we were going to crash hard.

Sierra was still hanging on behind me, but we were now headed up the street, right down the middle. The brick street we were now traveling down went straight ahead for about four blocks before coming to a *T*. It was not level. It sloped down toward both sides. At the end of the first block was a large drainage ditch where all the excess water ran off. My chair veered to the left toward the opening that led to the ditch.

In a matter of seconds, an endless number of possible outcomes flashed through my mind. The slope of the street caused my chair to veer sharply to the left, and before I knew it, we crashed into the side of my own van. It was a miracle. We were stopped, I was still in my chair, and Sierra was untouched! She was now convinced I wasn't April-fooling her, so she reached up and turned off my chair.

My footrests had absorbed the majority of the impact. As I looked around to assess the damages, I noticed my feet were sitting nicely on top of the running boards. My shoes didn't have a scuff on them. Sierra ran back to the youth center for help.

When I went back inside the building, I found Sierra and asked, "Where did you think I was taking you?"

She said, "I don't know. I thought you might have been taking me to my friend's house or something."

As I thought about Sierra's response, I realized she did not know where I was taking her, but she trusted me because she believed I had a place in mind. I immediately thought of those moments in my hospital room and that inner voice urging me to trust. The lesson for me was clear. I needed to trust God with my life like Sierra trusted me for a ride. I needed to remember He has places in mind, even when I don't know where He is taking me.

Justin – Live for God's Purposes, Not Just Your Own

Being in a wheelchair and working with kids was never in any of my life plans, but as time passed, I began to like the many new ways I had found to be useful. God was using me for purposes I never imagined, and I found it fulfilling.

A few minutes into a class I was teaching at Cherry Street, I asked Justin to read the Bible verse in Matthew 4:4 that says, "Man does not live on bread alone, but on every word that comes from the mouth of God." I was shocked when he read, "Man does not live to breed alone. . . ."

I started to correct him, but decided it was best not to draw attention to his mistake. The room was full of fourth- and fifth-graders, and I did not want to spend the next ten minutes teaching them about breeding. Inwardly I was laughing hysterically, but as he read on, the words seemed to be an exclamation mark on the end of a long lesson God had been teaching me. Satisfaction does not come from getting what we want physically; it comes from getting what we need spiritually.

I had always thought living out my dream and having a relationship with the right girl would fill the emptiness in my heart, but I was wrong. In giving up the things I wanted out of life in order to give of myself to children, I had received something in return that I had never had when all I lived for was my own purposes. I received the sense of satisfaction I had always longed for.

So as Justin read on that day, I realized his words were for me; there is more to life than just "to breed alone." Life is not about my getting everything I dreamed of; it's about my fulfilling God's purposes for my life.

Renee – Serve Others Joyfully and Willingly

Being paralyzed and being a youth minister, I required a lot of help from others to do my job. During the four years I worked in the small town of Fredonia, Kansas, I often relied on the kids. Over time I began to see that Renee was one teenager I could count on to help me do just about anything. Never did I ask her to do something and see her respond with anything but a smile . . . except one time.

We were at a weekend youth conference. It was early Saturday morning, and we were pressed for time. After my friend Kevin sat me in my wheelchair, I went outside our hotel room with the van keys on my armrest. My plan was to have one of the kids help me into the van while Kevin finished getting himself ready.

When Renee came out of her room and I saw that she was ready, I asked her to take my keys, unlock the van, and let the lift down. From the look on her face, you would have thought I had asked her to tear down the engine and reassemble it. She reluctantly took the keys and started towards the van. Her friend Tasha walked alongside her. It was obvious they did not want to open my van, and they were whispering back and forth.

I was surprised at Renee's seemingly bad attitude towards doing this simple task, because she was a great example of what a servant should be. She was a hard worker, she was one of only a few who consistently stayed to help clean up after meals, and she rarely complained. I had no idea what was wrong with her. Maybe she was having a bad day, or maybe I had done something to make her mad.

I watched as they carefully opened my van. Soon I discovered the reason for Renee's reluctance. She and her friend had put toothpaste on all the door handles. I had foiled their plan to initiate my friend.

I laugh every time I think of this story, but I am also reminded of the huge difference in the way people serve others. There are some people who are like Renee. You can ask them to do something for you, and they almost always do it with a smile. You can tell they really want to help, and they consider it a privilege. But there are also some people who are not like Renee, and they have a bad attitude towards serving. Sure, they might do the task, but they do it reluctantly, often making sure someone hears how much of an effort it was for them to do the good deed.

Through being paralyzed and needing to be served by others, I realized that I had learned how I should serve others. Being a good servant is all about attitude. It involves being humble and putting the needs of others ahead of our own. Philippians 2:5–7 says, "Your attitude should be the same as that of Christ Jesus: who, being in very nature God, did not consider equality with God something to be grasped, but made himself nothing, taking the very nature of a servant."

When I think of Renee, I'm reminded to serve others willingly with humility, a positive attitude, and a smile—never reluctantly.

Christian – Learn from Your Experiences

In the fall of 1999, I watched a little boy named Christian climb onto the monkey bars. He climbed up the ladder, grabbed a hold of the bars, and "monkeyed" across. When he reached the end, he let go of the bar above him without taking time to position his feet on the bar beneath him. As he let go, his feet slipped and he fell backwards over another bar, scraping his backbone. When he finally hit the ground, he turned and looked up at the bar in disgust. I could almost hear his thoughts: "That hurt. I'll never do that again."

At this point in my life, I was working full-time as a tutor and youth minister. My family had enabled me to live in my own house, and I was making enough money to be off Social Security. I had accomplished much since becoming paralyzed, but I had been pondering why some things in life have to hurt so badly.

As I watched Christian experience the pain from his fall, I realized there were a lot of things I'd done that I would never do again because they hurt or cost me something: diving without thinking of the consequences, trying to date two girls at once, hammering a nail into an electrical outlet. My list goes on. I also realized that if some things did not hurt, we would keep doing them over and over and might never learn from them.

Webster's defines an *experience* as "the fact or state of having been affected by or gained knowledge through direct observation or participation in events or in a particular activity." In my book, that means something happened, you either saw it or were directly involved in it, you were somehow affected by it, and you learned something from it. I found it interesting that the definition implies we are to gain knowledge through our experiences.

As time went on following my accident, I began to see that whether something is your fault, someone else's, or it just happened, painful experiences often serve important purposes. They give us knowledge that we can use to help ourselves or help others.

Sarah – Find Joy in the Simple Things

In the spring of 2005, two neighbor girls were playing next door with the kittens. MaKenzie, age seven, and Sarah, age six, were no strangers to the six-hundred block of South Malcolm. They knew who lived in every house, and they knew the name of every dog and cat on the block. They had never really ventured into my yard to talk to me, so I took this as my chance to befriend them.

They were wearing roller blades, and I knew if they had any reservations about being around a guy in a wheelchair, I could fix that by pulling them behind my chair. A few laps up and down my driveway and I was certain we would become buddies.

Somehow I went from being the "train engine" to the guy who was "it" in a game of tag. The girls were laughing and teasing me, saying, "You can't catch us! You can't catch us!" I decided that flattening one of these girls would not help me make friends with them, so I chased them on the driveway, knowing I would always be "it."

Playing with the girls and taking walks to the park became a daily ritual. There were countless wheelchair rides and more games of tag. Even after they learned I could not catch them, I still had to be "it." As summer turned to fall, our time outside diminished. Many of our games gave way to paints and colors and animal charades.

When Christmas came, Sarah brought me some drawings and a card she had made. They were not in an envelope. She had wrapped them with Christmas wrapping paper.

The card read, "Dear Kevin, you bring me great joy when you try to run over me. Merry Christmas. Love, Sarah."

As I read Sarah's words, I was reminded that it is the simple things in life that often bring the greatest joy.

Chapter 12

INFLUENTIAL PEOPLE AND EXPERIENCES

The life lessons associated with each story in the previous chapter served as powerful tools, helping me accept paralysis and find new meaning and purpose in life. As I began to write about these children, I realized God had been at work in my life long before I became paralyzed. It was almost as if He used the kids to put exclamation marks at the end of life-long lessons.

The more I began to reflect on influential people and experiences that had been etched into my mind, the more I saw how God had used them to give me some of the basic foundational virtues I needed in order to overcome the unexpected challenges I would face after becoming paralyzed.

Coach Williams

From the time I was old enough to walk, my dad had a basketball in my hands. As a result, I was a pretty good player. Honors and awards for winning free-throw contests covered my dresser. Throughout my six years in junior high and high school, I started every varsity basketball game and led the team in scoring.

If you were to ask the guys I played with, all of them would agree my favorite thing about playing basketball was to score points. I loved to shoot the ball. If it was a close game and the clock was winding down, I wanted the ball. I wanted to take the shot because I was confident in my abilities. I was competitive and loved to win, but also a little selfish.

Not only was I a little selfish in the game of basketball, but I was also a little selfish in life. I didn't understand there was more to life than my own wants and needs. I didn't understand the value in giving to others. God used my coach, Jeff Williams, to help me begin to see the need to become more unselfish.

Coach taught us that basketball is a team game, and so is life. We were not put here to simply go after the things we want. We were put here to love God and to love each other. Over and

109

over, Coach reminded us of that truth. He talked about being good citizens and giving of ourselves to help others.

Coach wanted us to be more than good basketball players. He wanted us to be good people—people who didn't just think of what they could achieve for themselves, but people who purposely went out of their way to make someone else's life better. He wanted us to give unselfishly in the game of basketball and in the game of life.

It seemed like a silly thing to talk about in the locker room, but he would sometimes ask, "What did you do today for someone else?" Each of us took turns answering. Many times I had trouble thinking of something to say. It was embarrassing to think I had spent all day at school around hundreds of people I called friends, but had been concerned about nothing except my own agenda.

In our final high school game, six seconds remained on the clock. We were down by one point. Coach called time-out and drew up the play. He looked at me and said, "Catch the inbounds pass, dribble downcourt as fast as you can, and look for an open man. Give it up, and it will come back to you."

The last thing I wanted to do was give up the opportunity to shoot the last shot. I dribbled downcourt and reluctantly passed the ball to the guy on my left. My hesitance gave the defender enough time to react, and he deflected the ball away from my teammate. Miraculously, just like Coach said, the ball came bouncing right back to me, and I was wide open ten feet from the basket. I shot the ball right before the buzzer sounded, but it bounced off the rim. We lost the game, and our senior season was over. I wondered if my reluctance to give up the ball had cost us the game.

At the time, I could not see anything good ever coming from that experience, but now I see it as part of a life-long lesson God gave me through the game of basketball to be unselfish. When I started giving up what I wanted in order to give my life to kids, I saw how God has a way of miraculously giving back to us when we simply give our lives to Him.

Old Bill

Coach Williams wasn't the only person God used to teach me a thing or two about looking beyond my own self to find meaning and purpose in life. He also used the closest neighbor to our farm, an eighty-year-old man named Bill Wiggans.

Bill's house was about one mile away from ours. He also farmed the land directly across the road from our house. When my sister, brother,

111

and I would be playing outside, we would see Bill on his red tractor, working in the fields. He was usually our best customer when we set up a lemonade stand.

About six months before I was paralyzed, Bill came to the fertilizer plant where I worked part-time. As I loaded his fertilizer wagon, he walked over to me, said hello, and proceeded to inform me that my spiritual life was the most important part of my life. We weren't having a spiritual conversation, nor had we ever before. He just felt compelled to give me this message.

I didn't disagree with Bill. I just shook my head yes and continued working. I was not sure how to respond. Here was a man who had basically lived the life I wanted to live. Why was he giving me advice about my spiritual life?

At nineteen, I thought life would last eighty-plus years, and I thought if I worked hard enough, I would die an old, happy man with everything I wanted. As I shared earlier in this book, I didn't want much: a farm, a wife, a house, a job, and a few kids. I knew Bill was right, but my plan was to live out my dream and then consider what God wanted. I saw God as my helper. I wanted Him to help me achieve my goals and get to the places I wanted to be, not tell me where to go or what to do with my life.

It never crossed my mind that giving my life to God could fill the emptiness I had as a young adult. Each day I would pray, "God, make me a better Christian and direct my life," because I knew I should; but I never took the time to do the things it took to become a better Christian, and I never seriously pursued trying to find out what God's purpose for my life might be. My mind was focused on living out my dream. I thought living my dream was what I needed to be truly happy and satisfied with my life.

As my dreams vanished, Bill's words never left me. They still run through my mind as if he said them yesterday. I'm not sure why he chose those words. Perhaps it was God speaking through Bill, giving me a warning. Perhaps if I had heeded his words and changed my life, I would not be paralyzed.

Perhaps I'll never know all the details until I arrive in heaven and God sits me on His knee. Perhaps then He'll explain His ability to intertwine His will with our freedom to make life choices, and I'll understand why He allowed certain things to happen as they did.

Perhaps God knew the only way I would sit still long enough to really listen to Him was to literally sit me still. Perhaps He knew my life story would be an inspiration and an encouragement to many. Perhaps He knew others would see His power at work through my weakness.

But perhaps I really won't even care why I had to endure these unwanted circumstances on earth because perhaps Romans 8:18 is true and "our present sufferings are not worth comparing with the glory that will be revealed in us."

Perhaps one day I'll find Old Bill and let him know how grateful I am to know my spiritual life is the most important part of my life.

Mom and Dad

As I watched the kids I worked with develop ways of looking at things, I often looked back on my own "programming." Contrary to my belief then, my parents were doing what they were supposed to be doing when they made me work instead of letting me sit around watching TV. When they taught me things I did not think I needed to know and disciplined me for acting inappropriately, they were instilling in me some basic ideas that formed the way I would think and behave. They were programming me, providing me with some basic operating instructions they wanted me to follow.

Both my parents had an active role in my upbringing. Mom taught us to do basic things like read, write, learn Bible verses, play games, and cook. Dad worked on the farm, taught math, and loved sports, so he was responsible for most of what we learned in those areas. I learned many things from them—some taught, some caught—but what I'm most grateful for is that they displayed qualities every parent should show their children: (1) They loved me unconditionally. (2) They wanted the best for me. (3) They were willing to make sacrifices for me. (4) They disciplined me when I needed it.

While looking back, I realized there was yet another element that went beyond the programming I received from influential people and events—the truths in God's Word. Like my parents, they served as cornerstones in my life, giving me strength and providing guidance.

As I studied the Bible, one particular truth stood out. It said God's love for us is a lot like the love a father has for his child. As I began to compare, sure enough, I found that several things I had observed about my parents were also true about God: (1) He loves me unconditionally. (2) He wants the best for me. (3) He is willing to make sacrifices for me. (4) He disciplines me when I need it.

Before I go further, let me clarify some things. I believe there are circumstances that are meant to be changed, but there are also circumstances meant to change us. I do not believe every unwanted circumstance is God's way of disciplining or changing us; however, I do believe we should always keep that possibility in mind. God wants to teach us many things about life, and often He uses unwanted circumstances to grab our attention.

Do I believe God caused me to become paralyzed as some form of punishment? No, it was my choice to dive off that dock. I do believe, however, He knew the choice I would make and that He allowed me to make it.

Not only do I believe He allowed me to make the choice, but I also believe He has allowed me to suffer the natural consequences of my own poor choice without intervening. Why? I don't know. God doesn't always give us the answers we seek. We can only trust that He knows what is best for us and that as a loving father, He cares more about our eternal comfort than our temporary comfort.

For me, it is both helpful and comforting to understand that God gave me a picture of His love in my parents. Their ultimate goal was not to punish me or make my life miserable; they wanted me to enjoy the gift of life they had given me. However, when they felt it was necessary, they disciplined me. Usually they would take away something I valued, make life uncomfortable for me, or allow me to experience the unpleasant outcomes of my own bad choices without intervening.

To us, this often seems unfair, but loving parents know what their children need and will not discipline them without a purpose in mind. I believe God is the same way. He is like a father who disciplines his children as he thinks best. God has a purpose in mind for everything He allows them to experience.

A Loving Father Disciplines His Children

They (our earthly fathers) disciplined us for a little while as they thought best; but God disciplines us for our good, in order that we may share in his holiness. No discipline seems pleasant at the time, but painful. Later on, however, it produces a harvest of righteousness and peace for those who have been trained by it.

—Hebrews 12:10–11

As a kid, one of my favorite things was to ride through the pasture and "help" Dad feed the cows. At five years old, I wasn't much help; but I thought I was, and I loved to tag along. One day when Dad stepped out of the green '74 Chevy to unload the hay, I noticed something interesting lying on the floorboard. Buried in the tools and dust was a glass tube containing several tiny colored balls. I loved balls, so I broke the tube to get them out.

When Dad climbed back in and saw what I had done to his antifreeze tester, he reached over, grabbed my little toy truck, and tossed it out the window. I'm not sure if he thought I had learned my lesson or if he was tired of hearing me cry, but when we reached the gate, he climbed out to shut it and returned holding my toy. He had only thrown it in the back. He had taken it away because he wanted me to learn to have respect for other people's things, but he had it in his mind all along to give it back.

I've thought of this simple story hundreds of times since becoming paralyzed, hoping God planned to give my physical abilities back after He was sure I had learned some lesson. I have no way of knowing God's intent, but I take comfort in knowing God is like a father who disciplines his children as he thinks best. If He has to allow some things to be taken away temporarily so that we make it to heaven or become more like Christ or fulfill His purposes, then I believe He will. To us, this often sounds unfair, but God knows when we reach the gate of heaven, we will get it all back.

Chapter 13

LIFE METAPHORS

Life Is Like a Puzzle

B ack in the days before PCs, cable TV, and PlayStations, baseball, hide-and-seek, and board games reigned supreme in the lives of kids. My favorite thing to do on rainy or snowy days was to break out the Monopoly game. Like a greedy tyrant, I slowly accumulated property and money from my younger sister. Occasionally Mom pried us away from the money and started us on a puzzle.

Puzzles were not my favorite pastime, but I searched and twisted and tried to fit the pieces together. It was often a challenge. The first step in puzzle building was always to set the box somewhere so we could see it at all times. Second, we looked for the pieces with flat edges. They were the easiest to figure out because they formed the outline of the picture. The ones with two flat edges were the real no-brainers. They had to go in the corners.

From there the individual pieces of the puzzle were more difficult to piece together. We searched for pieces that looked as if they belonged together because of shape or color. I remember the feeling of satisfaction and the sense of purpose when two pieces fit. Often though, we grabbed a piece and twisted it, turning it every way imaginable, only to fail to make it fit. Sometimes we found a piece that made several other pieces fall into place, but then there were always a few that seemed as if they just did not belong. At these times, we felt like giving up.

My experiences with puzzles compare to my experiences with life. People, events, and experiences are the individual pieces. God gives us a few corner pieces in His Word to start. He wants us to admit our need for Him, turn from our unbelief, accept His Son as the sacrifice for our sins, and live our lives continually striving to become more like Him. From there our puzzles become unique as God gives us unique gifts and allows us to have unique experiences.

At times the pieces of my life have been so perplexing. No matter how hard I searched or how many different ways I tried to twist and connect them with the other pieces, they just did not seem to fit. Discouraged, I felt like giving up.

Unlike a puzzle, the picture of my life is not conveniently printed on the outside of a box. I cannot always see how a piece fits into the grand design. From where I sit, I can see only a partially completed puzzle; however, God sees the top of the box. He knows how the pieces of my life fit together to make up the picture of my life. Given my position here on earth, I have decided to simply trust that God has drawn a beautiful picture.

Life Is a Recycling Process

The dirt road that ran by our farmhouse was hardly a haven for recyclable goods, but every few days my mom, my sister, and I searched the ditches for aluminum cans as we rode along on our bikes. Sometimes we filled our sacks. Sometimes we found only a few cans. Afterwards, we smashed the cans and added them to our pile in the garage, hoping to collect enough to sell.

As a kid, recycling cans meant nothing more to me than a way to make a few dollars. Now I see the recycling process at work everywhere, even in my life. God has taken me through a process of change in order to be reused for new purposes.

To recycle something means to make it ready for reuse. Some things can be reused without undergoing much of a change. Others must go through a process of change in order to be reused, often for a new purpose.

When aluminum arrives at the recycling plant, it is checked and sorted to determine composition and value. If the scrap is of unknown quality, the aluminum will first be passed through large magnets. Depending on the type of contamination present, some scrap must be further processed.

The aluminum is then loaded into a furnace and completely melted so it can be cast or processed into something new. It can be rolled into plates, sheets, or wafer-thin foils the thickness of a human hair. The rolling process changes the characteristics of the metal, making it less brittle and more ductile.

Just as we recycle aluminum cans, God often recycles us. He may use us over and over. Or, if necessary, He takes us through a series of changes that draw out our impurities, change our characteristics, and make us willing to be changed into something new. We can then fulfill a new purpose.

Life Is Like a Chocolate Chip Cookie

According to the doctors, I was twenty-one days late. According to me, I think I was born on the exact day God planned, August 28, 1971. I am reminded of the promise in Romans 8:28 every time I think of my birth date, 8-28, or see that it's 8:28 a.m. or p.m. I believe I was born on 8-28-1971 so that I would learn to love the promise in this verse: "And we know that in all things God works for the good of those who love him, who have been called according to his purpose" (Romans 8:28).

This promise reminds me of an experience I had as a child. One day while Mom was mixing ingredients for chocolate chip cookies, I ran through the kitchen, scooped a little dough out of the bowl, and ate it as fast as I could. Mom always let me have a little dough, but I had already exceeded my limit during the previous batch. I was surprised she didn't chase me down and whop me; instead, she just laughed. She hadn't finished putting in all the ingredients, and it left an awful taste in my mouth. Come to find out, she hadn't quite made it to the point where she added the sugar.

It is this mixture of good- and bad-tasting ingredients that causes me to compare life to a chocolate chip cookie. The individual ingredients of a cookie are similar to the individual events in our lives. Some are good and leave a sweet taste. Others, like flour, baking powder, and raw eggs, leave a bad taste in our mouths if eaten separately. If we didn't know things like flour and baking powder have a purpose within the overall plan and are important parts of the cookie-making process, we certainly would not want to put them into a cookie. But when Mom takes those bad-tasting ingredients, throws in some good-tasting ingredients, mixes them, and bakes them according to her plan (recipe), the end result is something good.

In life, many things do not seem to belong to our version of the recipe, and we have no idea how God could use them for anything good. But according to Romans 8:28, God can take the bad-tasting experiences, throw in some good-tasting experiences, mix them all together, bake them according to His plan, and make everything end up good according to His purposes.

Each day I try to operate on the "cookie principle" in Romans 8:28 and trust God will somehow mix all the individual ingredients of my life together to make it all turn out good in the end. The key to doing this is to understand that God's purposes are not our purposes. Romans 8:28 says all things work together for good according to *His* purposes, not ours.

Life Is a Game

One day at Cherry Street, I told my class of fourth-grade boys that we were going to play a game. They were excited. I didn't normally start Bible study with a game. We had been talking about the fact that God has two general purposes for us:

1. That we make it to heaven
2. That we spend our time on earth becoming more like Christ

It seemed as if the kids were not all that interested, so I divided them into two teams. My helper put a Ping-Pong ball on the table, and without giving them any rules or a goal, I said, "Go."

Some of the boys tried to knock the ball away from the others. Some tried to gain possession of it. Some watched quietly from their chairs. After a few seconds of complete chaos, one of the boys looked up at me and said, "What game are we playing?" By this time, one boy was stretched out on the floor with his entire body over the ball. It looked like he was recovering a fumble. I stopped the game and had everyone listen to the boy's question, "What game are we playing?"

This was the question I had hoped someone would ask. I stopped the game and said, "When we do not know the purpose of a game, it's confusing and it seems pointless." I told them the rules and the purpose of the game, and we played again. This time everyone knew what to do in order to help their team win because they knew the purpose of the game.

Life is like a game. God has put us here on earth with others, given us many things, and told us to live. Sadly, many of us go through life not knowing our purpose. We wander aimlessly, unsure of how to play the game. We make up our own rules, trying to do the best we can to figure it out.

At some point, we need to look to the One who started the game and ask the question, "What game are we playing?"

Fortunately, we don't have to look too far past Romans 8:28 to find an answer. In Romans 8:29, God tells us we have an awesome destiny: to be like Christ. "For those God foreknew he also predestined to be conformed to the image of his Son." This clearly states that one of God's purposes for His children is that they become more like Christ.

If we learn this and make it our goal as well, we will know how to play the game of life, our lives will never lack for meaning despite our circumstances, and we will be rewarded in the end with a win.

Life Is a Race

Let us run with perseverance the race marked out for us, fixing our eyes on Jesus, the pioneer and perfecter of faith. For the joy set before him he endured the cross.

—Hebrews 12:1–2

I love metaphors. Forrest Gump had a good one: "Life is like a box of chocolates; you never know what you are going to get." Joe Dirt's wasn't bad: "Life's a garden—dig it." The apostle Paul had a good one, too. He said life is like a race that has been marked out for us to run.

During my sophomore year in high school, I ran the 800-meter and the 3200-meter relay. I wasn't quite fast enough to win the 800, but our relay team set the school record. I thought I had enough endurance, so I told my coach I wanted to run the individual 3200-meter race. The first time I ran it, I placed sixth with a time of ten minutes and fifty seconds. The next meet, I had hopes of doing better, but as I started around the track, my back began to hurt. With each step, it hurt a little more, but I was determined to stick it out. The reward at the end was worth the pain.

127

By the end of the fourth lap, my back was killing me and I wanted to quit; however, I was still in third place, and the leaders were just a few strides ahead. I endured one more lap because third place could still win a medal. As I approached the first curve in the sixth lap, another runner flew by me. The distance between us increased. I knew I would never be able to catch up. Reluctantly I swallowed my pride, stepped off the track, laid on my back, and did not move.

In every race, and in life, there is a predetermined course and an end to be attained. Hebrews 12 compares our life to a race and gives us some insight on how to run it. First it says we are to run with perseverance. To persevere means to persist with a purpose. A purpose is an end to be attained. God's end goal is to reward us with eternal life in heaven.

While we are here on earth, I believe God has also planned individual races for us to run. He has thought about what He would like us to do with our lives, and He has given us gifts, talents, passions, and experiences that we can use in unique ways. Ephesians 2:10 reminds us, "For we are God's handiwork, created in Christ Jesus to do good works, which God prepared in advance for us to do."

Hebrews 12 goes on to say we should fix our eyes on Jesus while running our race. This means we should keep our focus on Jesus. Why Jesus? He is both our reward and our example. He wrote the book, if you will, on running His race with perseverance. He looked beyond the struggle and pain He endured while running His race and kept His focus on the end goal. He did not give up, even in the darkest hours.

How did He keep from giving up? In John 6:38, Jesus indicated that He knew His race was marked out for Him by His Father. He said, "For I have come down from heaven not to do my will but to do the will of him who sent me." He knew there was an end to be attained through both His life and His death. He focused more on the joy set before Him than the suffering around Him.

As I learned from my track days, rewards have an amazing influence on a person's willingness to persevere. As long as I had the hope of being rewarded, I was willing to endure great pain. Once that hope was gone, so was my willingness to continue running the race.

Fortunately, the hope of reward that we have in Christ cannot be taken from us. When things happen that make us feel like quitting the race, it's important we take a page out of Jesus' play-book. We need to focus on the right thing—the finish line. Unlike a runner who falls into fourth place and loses all hope of being rewarded in the end, we have God's promise that we will never be without hope of reward when we are running the race He has marked out for us.

Life Is Embroidery

> *Have you not known? Have you not heard? Has it not been told you from the beginning? Have you not understood from the foundations of the earth? It is He who sits above the circle of the earth, and its inhabitants are like grasshoppers, who stretches out the heavens like a curtain, and spreads them out like a tent to dwell in.*
> —Isaiah 40:21–23 NKJV

The story is told about a boy whose mother used to embroider. The boy sat at her knee, looked up from the floor, and asked, "What are you doing?"

She replied, "I am embroidering."

From the underside, he watched her work within the boundaries of the little round hoop she held. He wondered why she was using some dark threads along with the bright ones and why they seemed so jumbled from his point of view.

"It sure looks messy from where I am," he complained.

She smiled, looked down, and gently said, "My son, you go about your playing for a while, and when I am finished with my embroidering, I will put you on my knee and let you see it from my side."

When his mother called him, he was surprised to see a beautiful sunset. He could not believe it, because from underneath it had looked so messy. Then his mother said, "From underneath it did look messy and jumbled, but you could not see the plan on top. Now, when you look at it from my side, you can see what I was doing."

From where we sit here on earth and underneath the heavens, our view of God's overall plan is limited. We will never be able to see everything God sees because we are positioned here on earth. We do not have the luxury of knowing how certain events or circumstances will play out. From our perspective, the events in our lives often look like jumbled, messy events.

One day God will sit us on His knee and show us the view from His side. For now, we must trust that God will turn what seems jumbled and messy into something beautiful.

Chapter 14

UNWANTED
CIRCUMSTANCES

L ooking back, I realize I didn't just wake up one day and feel like I had reached some magical point where I fully accepted my paralysis. In fact, twenty-some years later, I have days where I'm extremely frustrated because of my limitations. It's not how I want to live. At times I feel as if I have to accept it all over again, because I'm faced with paralysis when I wake up each morning. On occasion I find myself discouraged, asking God why He allows me to suffer day after day.

Learning to "live with it" is an ongoing, daily struggle, but God has given me some basic truths about unwanted circumstances that have become a real help. The truths I share in this chapter weren't put together by a theologian; they are simply truths I've observed and found helpful. I hope they are helpful to you also.

Unwanted Circumstances Cannot Rob Life of Meaning

Dr. Viktor Frankl, a concentration camp survivor, wrote a book called *Man's Search for Meaning*. In it he expresses that the deepest need we have is to find meaning or a potential meaning in life and its happenings. His deepest experience was in Auschwitz. The odds of surviving there were 1 in 28.

Dr. Frankl had written about his experiences and thoughts and had hoped if he did not survive, at least his writings would. After entering the camp, however, prisoners were stripped of every possession and given the worn-out rags of gassed inmates. His book, tucked inside his coat pocket, was taken. It seemed to him that death was imminent.

It was under these circumstances that Dr. Frankl wondered whether his life was now void of meaning. His concern in this situation was not like his comrades. They were thinking, "Will we survive the camp? If not, all this suffering has no meaning." He was thinking, "Has all this suffering, this dying around us, a meaning? If not, then ultimately there is no meaning to survival; for a life whose meaning depends upon such a happenstance—as whether one escapes or not—ultimately would not be worth living at all."[1]

In many ways, being confined to a wheelchair and told I would never walk again was like being put into a prison and told I would never escape. Over time I saw that if my life had no meaning while I was paralyzed, then neither would it have meaning if I was healed. Like Dr. Frankl, I also concluded that a life whose meaning was dependent upon such a happenstance—as whether one is healed or not—would not be worth living at all.

Unwanted Circumstances Do Not Indicate God Does Not Love Us

Like most people who experience an unwanted circumstance where they suffer some sort of loss, I was bitter and upset that my heavenly Father had allowed it. I could not see how anything good could possibly come from it. I was overwhelmed with loss and disappointment. I spent countless hours trying to figure out whether I was being disciplined, whether I was just suffering from my own poor choice, whether Satan was trying to destroy my life, or whether it was a combination of all the above.

The more I thought about it, the more frustrated I became. I even found myself wondering if God still loved me and cared about me. The truth of the matter is, everyone who has ever lived (even Jesus) experiences unwanted circumstances. It's a part of life. I believe Jesus understood this. I also believe He understood that in order to fulfill His God-given purpose, He would have to face the unwanted circumstances head-on.

Before being arrested and crucified, Jesus took His disciples to a place called Gethsemane, and He said to them, "Stay here while I pray." Going a little farther, he fell with his face to the ground and prayed, "My Father, if it is possible, may this cup be taken from Me. Yet not as I will, but as You will." Then He returned to His disciples and found them sleeping.

He went away a second time and prayed, "My Father, if it is not possible for this cup to be taken away unless I drink it, may Your will be done." When He came back, He again found them sleeping, because their eyes were heavy. So He left them and went away once more and prayed the third time, saying the same thing (see Matthew 26:38–44).

Jesus knew the suffering and death He was about to experience was not going to be pleasant. He was filled with sorrow and anguish. Instead of calling on the Father to send twelve legions of angels to rescue Him, Jesus accepted being arrested, beaten, and crucified.

Like Jesus, we often find ourselves in situations that are hard to accept, asking the Father to take it from us if it is possible. This does not mean we should sulk and conclude that God does not love us. We need to follow Jesus' example. We need to remember that everyone faces unwanted circumstances and then strive to reach the place where we care more about God's purposes being accomplished in our lives than we do our own comfort.

Unwanted Circumstances Create Opportunities for God to Show His Power

Someone once told me God allows problems into our lives for one of several reasons: to inspect us, to correct us, to direct us, to perfect us, or to protect us. I think sometimes it is all five reasons, but I'm not God, so I can't say what is true for each and every person in each and every circumstance. When I look at my own life and the examples given in the Bible, I think it's pretty clear; God can and does use all types of unwanted circumstances to work in the lives of His children.

In John 9:1–3, it says that as Jesus went along, he saw a man blind from birth. His disciples asked him, "Rabbi, who sinned, this man or his parents, that he was born blind?" Jesus replied by saying, "Neither this man nor his parents sinned, but this happened so that the works of God might be displayed in him." Jesus then healed the man from his blindness, and all the people who knew him were amazed.

In this story, we see a man who had to live with an unwanted circumstance. He lived every day of his life being blind. We see parents who lived with the pain of watching their child suffer every day. They had probably asked a host of questions that began with *why*, only to receive no definite answers. They most likely saw the suffering as the disciples did: as a punishment for some sin.

After many long years of the man's suffering, Jesus gave them an unexpected answer to their questions right before healing the man. He said it was not anyone's fault, nor was it a punishment. God allowed the man to be born blind so that He would have an opportunity to show His power to the world.

Once when Paul was in a situation he did not like, he asked God three times to change it. Instead of granting Paul's request, God said, " 'My grace is sufficient for you, for My strength is made perfect in weakness.' Therefore most gladly

I will rather boast in my infirmities, that the power of Christ may rest upon me" (2 Corinthians 12:9, NKJV).

Basically, God was telling Paul the same thing my little brother told me: "Live with it." Only God's answer was accompanied with a declaration that through Paul's weakness, God would somehow show His power. Paul did not know exactly how God would work, and it wasn't the response he wanted from God, but knowing God had a reason for allowing the unwanted circumstance gave Paul what he needed to accept it.

Often God shows His strength by changing circumstances, as He did for the blind man. At other times, He gives us the inner strength to accept an unwanted, unchangeable circumstance, as He did for Paul. Either way, unwanted circumstances are opportunities for God to work and to show His strength.

Knowing God might have a reason for allowing me to experience paralysis, even if it was not to heal me, gave me a sense of meaning and purpose. It gave me something to hope for. It was exactly what I needed to help me accept paralysis, and it increased my desire to continue living life to the fullest, because I knew God could use my unwanted circumstances to show His power, no matter the outcome.

Unwanted Circumstances Present Opportunities For Our Faith to Grow

> *In this [the salvation God gave through Jesus Christ] you greatly rejoice, though now for a little while, if need be, you have been grieved by various trials, that the genuineness of your faith, being much more precious than gold that perishes, though it is tested by fire, may be found to praise, honor, and glory at the revelation of Jesus Christ.*
>
> —1 Peter 1:6–7 NKJV

Often I will ask kids, "What is the most valuable thing you have?" Then I'll ask, "What would God say is the most valuable thing you have?" I receive all kinds of answers, but I think God would say the most valuable thing we possess is our faith.

I say this because in 1 Peter 1:6–7, Peter says our faith is more valuable than the most precious metal on earth, gold. This is particularly interesting to me as I look back on an incident in Peter's life that likely contributed to his way of thinking.

It's Passover. Jesus and the disciples are sitting around a table, talking. A lot of big things are about to happen. Jesus is about to be betrayed

139

by Judas, denied by Peter, and arrested by the Roman soldiers. The disciples are likely floating on cloud nine, clueless of what is to come. They have spent the last three years as Jesus' most devoted followers, and Jesus had just told them they were going to be appointed a high place in His kingdom. They probably felt as if Jesus was rewarding them for their dedication.

But then, in Luke 22:31–32, Jesus singles out Peter and tells him he is about to go through an experience that will shake and almost destroy his faith. Jesus says, "Simon, Simon! Indeed, Satan has asked for you, that he may sift you as wheat. But I have prayed for you, that your faith should not fail; and when you have returned to Me, strengthen your brethren" (NKJV).

Jesus compares Peter's upcoming experience to the process of sifting wheat, a process where piles of grain were shoveled onto a sifter, or sieve, typically a four-by-four-feet wooden frame with a screened bottom, then shaken vigorously. All the dirt and chaff would fall through the screen to the ground. When the shaking was complete, only the pure kernels of grain remained.

This bothered me at first. Why would Jesus allow Peter to go through this experience? It appears obvious Satan had to ask permission to do this. If I were Peter and the devil wanted to shake my faith hard in hopes that I'd fall away from Jesus like chaff, I would want Jesus to say, "Satan has asked to sift you as wheat, but I told him he couldn't touch you." Jesus didn't do that; instead, He told Peter that He had prayed for his faith, that it would not fail.

Why did Jesus single out Peter's faith? I believe the reason is that Jesus was more concerned with Peter's faith than He was with any other aspect of Peter's life.

This experience was likely the reason Peter could confidently write, "If need be, you have been grieved by various trials, that the genuineness of your faith, being much more precious than gold that perishes, though it is tested by fire, may be found to praise, honor, and glory at the revelation of Jesus Christ."

Peter had learned, firsthand, the value system of God. He had learned that God was more concerned with his faith than with anything else. God knew the unwanted circumstance was ultimately going to benefit Peter by causing his faith to be purified and to grow stronger. But that wasn't the only thing God had in mind by allowing Peter to be sifted. Jesus told Peter that the end result of his experience was not only for the benefit of Peter's faith, but it was also going to be used to strengthen the faith of others.

Until I understood that God was more concerned with my faith than with me getting everything I wanted in life, my trials seemed like a meaningless series of disappointments. When I saw that trials developed my faith and could impact the faith of those around me, it gave my trials meaning. It's not that I began to enjoy my unwanted circumstances, but I just saw there might be a higher purpose. God might want to use it for my benefit or to benefit those around me.

Unwanted Circumstances Show Us Our Need for God

Over the course of the last twenty years, I've been fortunate to see God at work doing many things through my accident. Knowing God has used me and my paralysis to influence and encourage others has made life easier.

But I've met people with tragic stories far worse than mine. I've witnessed events where it was difficult, if not impossible, to see anything good come from the unwanted circumstance. I've seen a teenager's life cut short by a senseless tragedy. I've seen a young, healthy father and husband die suddenly for no apparent reason. I've listened to people tell stories of being diagnosed with terminal illnesses and given a limited number of days to live. I watched my grandmother suffer through cancer, diabetes, and then Alzheimer's. She lived for months not knowing who we were or where she was. She had no quality of life. It was hard to understand what purpose God had for her to remain alive.

When I see these types of things happen, I almost always wonder why God allows it and how He might use it. Often I come up with no answers. Maybe there is no other reason except to show us we need God. Maybe God uses these types of things to remind us how fragile life is, to cause us to long for something this life cannot offer and no person or circumstance can ever take away.

Unwanted Circumstances Create Opportunities for Us to Respond

Unwanted circumstances often come upon us unexpectedly, causing us to become angry and bitter towards God and others, but God can use unwanted circumstances to accomplish many things. They cause us to do things we might not otherwise do. They open and close doors, cause us to realign our priorities, and lead us to serve in ways we never thought possible. They bring out gifts and qualities we never knew we had. They develop character traits. They cause us to make decisions. They force us to respond. Our response can then alter the course of our life.

In many cases, I believe our response to our circumstance is even more important than the circumstance itself. Obviously, it would not be possible to respond to a circumstance that did not exist, but as far as how it impacts the course of our life, I believe that our response to our circumstance is just as important, if not more important, than the circumstance itself.

When Moses led the Israelites out of Egypt and arrived at the place God had prepared for them, the Lord said to him, "Send some men to explore the land of Canaan, which I am giving to the Israelites" (Numbers 13:2). So Moses sent twelve spies into the land to see what it was like.

Ten came back saying, "We went into the land to which you sent us, and it does flow with milk and honey! Here is its fruit. But the people who live there are powerful, and the cities are fortified and very large. . . . We can't attack those people; they are stronger than we are. All the people we saw there are of great size. . . . We seemed like grasshoppers in our own eyes, and we looked the same to them" (Numbers 13:27–33).

Joshua and Caleb returned and said, "The land we passed through and explored is exceedingly good. If the LORD is pleased with us, he will lead us into that land, a land flowing with milk and honey, and will give it to us. Only do not rebel against the LORD. And do not be afraid of the people of the land, because we will swallow them up. Their protection is gone, but the LORD is with us. Do not be afraid of them" (Numbers 14:7–9).

In this story, we see that the circumstances the Israelites faced forced them to make a choice. God purposely put them in a position where they had to respond to their circumstances. Everyone knew God had promised them the land, and everyone saw the same obstacles they would have to overcome; but not everyone had the same response. Caleb and Joshua said, "We can do this. Let's go." The rest said, "We cannot do this. Let's go back."

The negative report from the ten men spread throughout the camp. The Israelite people began to operate on the faulty assumption that God had brought them this far only to let them be defeated by their enemies. Granted, the people they had to fight were bigger and stronger, but God had already promised to give them the land. All they had to do was trust God and go into the land to take possession of it.

Because of their response to the situation they were in, they spent the next forty years barely surviving in the desert. Had they been able to see beyond the physical obstacles and focus on the things God had promised, they could have been really living in the place God had prepared for them.

From this story, it's easy to see how circumstances cause us to make decisions we wouldn't otherwise have to make. They present opportunities for us to respond positively in faith by choosing to trust God. They also present opportunities for us to respond negatively by choosing not to trust God.

We can also see how our decision to respond negatively or positively to our circumstances can make a huge difference. Like the ten spies with the negative report, we often let our feelings of fear, failure, disappointment, loss, and uncertainty overwhelm us and overcome us. We become so focused on the obstacles we face that instead of overcoming them, we see them as too big or too hard to overcome. As a result, we fail to respond positively. We give up.

After the forty-year period, only Joshua and Caleb were allowed to enter the land God had prepared for them. The only difference between them and the other ten spies was their response to their circumstances.

Chapter 15

THE END

God did not change my circumstances like I had hoped; instead, He changed me.

The hardest part about writing this book has been deciding how to end it. I've written and rewritten countless possibilities. I have found myself telling God how great it would be to end this book with a chapter describing how my spinal cord had been miraculously healed. I've pointed out to God how much glory He would receive by allowing me to walk again. I have prayed, "God, if only I was healed, think of how many people would believe in You. Think of all the things I could do for others. Instead of me needing help, I could help others."

While playing out the different scenarios in my mind, I began to wonder. Does God receive more glory for changing a circumstance or for changing a person?

I suppose there is not a clear-cut answer for every circumstance, and we really have no way of measuring the amount of glory God receives from any of His works. Ultimately, what matters is that we decide to allow God to receive glory regardless of how He chooses to work. For years, however, I believed God would get more glory from changing my circumstance than from changing me.

I'm not so sure anymore. You see, a physical healing would've lasted only forty, fifty, sixty years until my body quit working again. Instead, God chose to do a work in me that will last forever.

Through my accident, He taught me to see life as a fragile gift that can be gone in an instant. I learned to see the small things as big things. Things like family and friends, breathing, talking, feeling the warmth of the sun, thinking, and seeing became treasured gifts. When I left the hospital and ventured back out into the real world, God continued to change my way of looking at life.

God taught me to learn to live with my unwanted circumstances and to learn from my experiences. He urged me to trust in Him when I had no idea where He was leading me. He challenged me to give up my own hopes and dreams to give of myself to others. He taught me to look for new ways to be useful.

Through my needing to be served, He showed me how to be a servant. He showed me how simple things often bring others the greatest joy and that giving what you have to give is more important than what you have to give.

He taught me to be unselfish. He showed me that my spiritual life is the most important part of my life and that He cares more about our eternal comfort than our temporary comfort here on earth.

Sometimes I wish I would have learned these things some other way. It would've been nice if I could've read a book by someone who had these experiences and learned from them. But would I have listened? Would I have really learned these truths and made them an integral part of my life? It's impossible to know for sure, but I'm guessing *no*.

The way it happened made the life lessons personal. It was as if God was there all along the way, teaching, guiding, and working in all things to bring about good. I believe He's allowed me to have these experiences so that I could learn and then share them with others.

So, back to my question, would God have received more glory from changing my circumstance than from changing me? I still don't know for sure, but I don't think so.

As I was finishing this book, my pastor shared a thought with me. He said, "God is most glorified in us when we are most satisfied in Him." I think that pretty much sums up what I've learned. Life is full of unwanted circumstances, problems, and obstacles. When I jump over one hurdle or climb one mountain, I can expect another to come; however, I must learn to be satisfied in God regardless of my circumstances.

My challenge to you is this: Don't allow unwanted circumstances to make you bitter—use them to make you better. Don't let them defeat you—use them to develop you. Allow God to work in your life despite unwanted circumstances. Sure, strive to change the unwanted circumstances that you can, but remember, when God doesn't change a circumstance, you just have to take the advice of that wise three-year-old brother of mine and learn to *live with it.*

PHOTOS

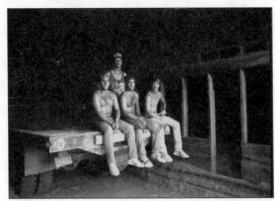

Pictured sitting on the hay truck are Trent Schell, Kevin Olson, and Jerrod Richards. Standing is Rob McMillen.

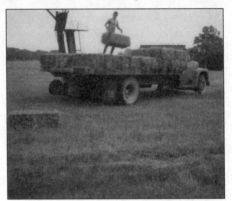

Hauling hay on my grandpa's farm

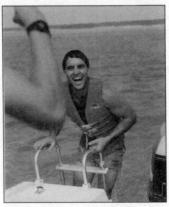

Climbing into the boat after a fun day of skiing

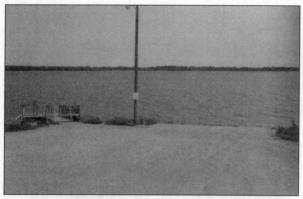

Boat dock and ramp where my accident took place

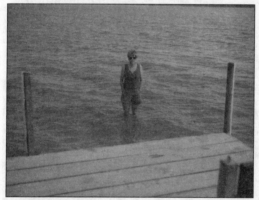

*My Aunt Pat standing near the dock,
showing the depth of the water*

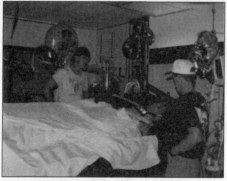

*Jerrod Richards and Stan Lopeman visiting me at the
University of Kansas Medical Center*

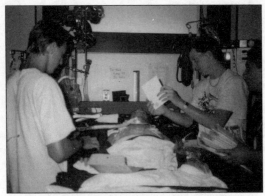

*Kevin Cooper, Doug Hutton, and Robert
DelaTorre reading birthday cards*

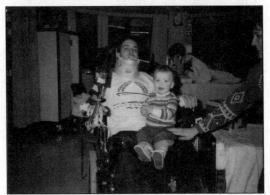

My youngest brother, James, visiting me at Craig Hospital

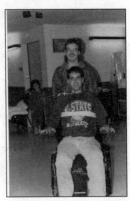

Brad and I at Craig Hospital

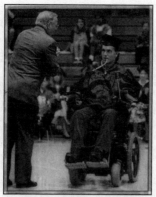

Graduating from Neosho County Community College

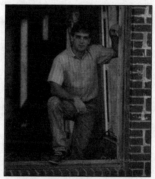

Senior picture, 1989

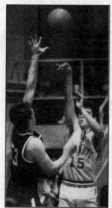

Showing off my jump shot

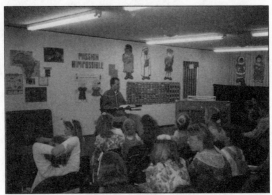

*Speaking to a group of kids at a local church
shortly after being released from the hospital*

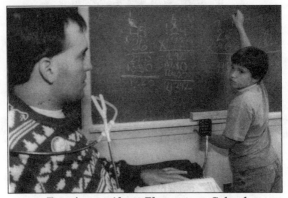

Tutoring at Alcott Elementary School

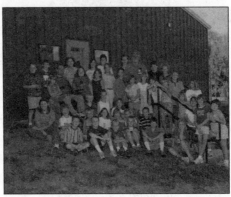

Our Cherry Street Youth Center kids

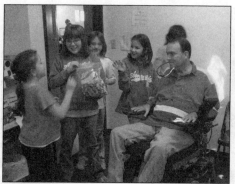

*At Cherry Street Youth Center rewarding
kids for memorizing Bible verses*

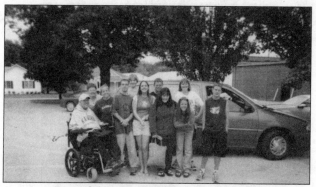

*Part of the youth group from Fredonia
preparing to leave for a trip*

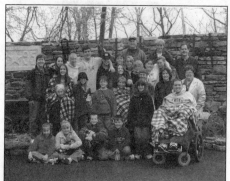

*More of the youth group at Young Christians
Weekend in Branson, Missouri*

157

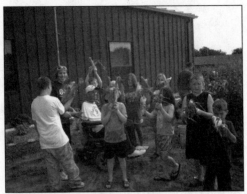

*Cherry Street Youth Center kids in the
garden showing off the corn they grew*

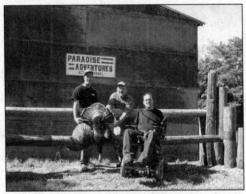

*Steve Hanna, Kurt Nunnenkamp, and I proudly displaying
the turkey I shot at Paradise Adventures*

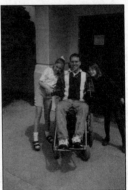

*Miranda and a friend hanging out
with me at recess*

158

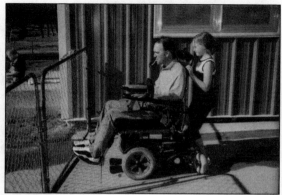

*Cherry Street Youth Center kid finishing up
a ride on my wheelchair*

Notes

1. Victor E. Frankl, *Man's Search for Meaning: An
Introduction to Logotherapy* (New York: Simon &
Schuster, Inc., 1984), 118-119.